Allyn and Bacon

Quick Guide to the Internet for Health

1999 Edition

Michael Olpin
Concord College

Doug Gotthoffer
California State University–Northridge

Allyn and Bacon
Boston • London • Toronto • Sydney • Tokyo • Singapore

Vice President and Director, Allyn and Bacon Interactive: Kevin B. Stone
Multimedia Editor: Marnie S. Greenhut
Editorial Production Administrator, Media: Robert Tonner
Cover Designer: Jennifer Hart
Editorial Production Service: Omegatype Typography, Inc.

NOTICE: Between the time web site information is gathered and then published it is not unusual for some sites to have closed. Also, the transcription of URLs can result in unintended typographical errors. The publisher would appreciate notification where these occcur so that they may be corrected in subsequent editions. Thank you.

TRADEMARK CREDITS: Where information was available, trademarks and registered trademarks are indicated below. When detailed information was not available, the publisher has indicated trademark status with an initial capital where those names appear in the text.

Macintosh is a registered trademark of Apple Computer, Inc.

Microsoft is a registered trademark of Microsoft Corporation. Windows, Windows95, and Microsoft Internet Explorer are trademarks of Microsoft Corporation.

Netscape and the Netscape Navigator logo are registered trademarks of Netscape Communications Corporation.

ISBN 0-205-29570-3

Printed in the United States of America

10 9 8 7 6 5 4 3 2 1   01 00 99 98

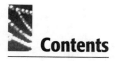

Contents

Introduction to the Internet

You're about to embark on an exciting experience as you become one of the millions of citizens of the Internet. In spite of what you might have heard, the Internet can be mastered by ordinary people before they earn a college degree and even if they're not majoring in rocket science.

Some Things You Ought to Know

Much of the confusion over the Internet comes from two sources. One is terminology. Just as the career you're preparing for has its own special vocabulary, so does the Internet. You'd be hard pressed to join in the shoptalk of archeologists, librarians, or carpenters if you didn't speak their language. Don't expect to plop yourself down in the middle of the Internet without some buzzwords under your belt, either.

The second source of confusion is that there are often many ways to accomplish the same ends on the Internet. This is a direct by-product of the freedom so highly cherished by Net citizens. When someone has an idea for doing something, he or she puts it out there and lets the Internet community decide its merits. As a result, it's difficult to put down in writing the *one exact* way to send email or find information on slugs or whatever.

Most of the material you'll encounter in this book applies to programs that run on the Macintosh computer. If you own or use a PC, you'll discover there are some cosmetic and technical differences. On the other hand, both computers offer the same major functionality. What you can do on the Mac you can usually do on the PC, and vice versa. If you can't find a particular command or function mentioned in the book on your computer, chances are it's there, but in a different place or with a slightly different name. Check the manual or online help that came with your computer, or ask a more computer-savvy friend or professor.

And relax. Getting up to speed on the Internet takes a little time, but the effort will be well rewarded. Approach learning your way around the Internet with the same enthusiasm and curiosity you approach learning your way around a new college campus. This isn't a competition. Nobody's keeping score. And the only winner will be you.

In *Understanding Media,* Marshall McLuhan presaged the existence of the Internet when he described electronic media as an extension of our central nervous system. On the other hand, today's students introduced to the Internet for the first time describe it as "Way cool."

No matter which description you favor, you are immersed in a period in our culture that is transforming the way we live by transforming the nature of the information we live by. As recently as 1980, intelligence was marked by "knowing things." If you were born in that year, by the time you were old enough to cross the street by yourself, that definition had changed radically. Today, in a revolution that makes McLuhan's vision tangible, events, facts, rumors, and gossip are distributed instantly to all parts of the global body. The effects are equivalent to a shot of electronic adrenaline. No longer the domain of the privileged few, information is shared by all the inhabitants of McLuhan's global village. Meanwhile, the concept of information as intelligence feels as archaic as a television remote control with a wire on it (ask your parents about that).

With hardly more effort than it takes to rub your eyes open in the morning you can connect with the latest news, with gossip about your favorite music group or TV star, with the best places to eat on spring break, with the weather back home, or with the trials and tribulations of that soap opera character whose life conflicts with your history class.

You can not only carry on a real-time conversation with your best friend at a college half a continent away you can see and hear her, too. Or, you can play interactive games with a dozen or more world-wide, world-class, challengers; and that's just for fun.

When it comes to your education, the Internet has shifted the focus from amassing information to putting that information to use. Newspaper and magazine archives are now almost instantly available, as are the contents of many reference books. Distant and seemingly unapproachable, experts are found answering questions in discussion groups or in electronic newsletters.

The Internet also addresses the major problem facing all of us in our split-second, efficiency-rated culture: Where do we find the time? The

part

1

Internet allows professors and students to keep in touch, to collaborate and learn, without placing unreasonable demands on individual schedules. Professors are posting everything from course syllabi to homework solutions on the Internet, and are increasingly answering questions online, all in an effort to ease the pressure for face-to-face meetings by supplementing them with cyberspace offices. The Internet enables students and professors to expand office hours into a twenty-four-hour-a-day, seven-day-a-week operation. Many classes have individual sites at which enrolled students can gather electronically to swap theories, ideas, resources, gripes, and triumphs.

By freeing us from some of the more mundane operations of information gathering, and by sharpening our information-gathering skills in other areas, the Internet encourages us to be more creative and imaginative. Instead of devoting most of our time to gathering information and precious little to analyzing and synthesizing it, the Internet tips the balance in favor of the skills that separate us from silicon chips. Other Internet citizens can gain the same advantage, however, and as much as the Internet ties us together, it simultaneously emphasizes our individual skills—our ability to connect information in new, meaningful, and exciting ways. Rarely have we had the opportunity to make connections and observations on such a wide range of topics, to create more individual belief systems, and to chart a path through learning that makes information personally useful and meaningful.

part
1

A Brief History of the Internet

The 20th century's greatest advance in personal communication and freedom of expression began as a tool for national defense. In the mid-1960s, the Department of Defense was searching for an information analogy to the new Interstate Highway System, a way to move computations and computing resources around the country in the event the Cold War caught fire. The immediate predicament, however, had to do with the Defense Department's budget, and the millions of dollars spent on computer research at universities and think tanks. Much of these millions was spent on acquiring, building, or modifying large computer systems to meet the demands of the emerging fields of computer graphics, artificial intelligence, and multiprocessing (where one computer was shared among dozens of different tasks).

While this research was distributed across the country, the unwieldy, often temperamental, computers were not. Though researchers at MIT had spare time on their computer, short of packing up their notes and traveling to Massachusetts, researchers at Berkeley had no way to use it. Instead, Berkeley computer scientists would wind up duplicating MIT hardware in California. Wary of being accused of re-inventing the wheel, the Advanced Research Projects Agency (ARPA), the funding arm of the Defense Department, invested in the ARPANET, a private network that would allow disparate computer systems to communicate with each other. Researchers could remain ensconced among their colleagues at their home campuses while using computing resources at government research sites thousands of miles away.

A small cadre of ARPANET citizens soon began writing computer programs to perform little tasks across the Internet. Most of these programs, while ostensibly meeting immediate research needs, were written for the challenge of writing them. These programmers, for example, created the first email systems. They also created games like Space Wars and Adventure. Driven in large part by the novelty and practicality of email, businesses and institutions accepting government research funds begged and borrowed their way onto the ARPANET, and the number of connections swelled.

As the innocence of the 1960s gave way the business sense of the 1980s, the government eased out of the networking business, turning the ARPANET (now Internet) over to its users. While we capitalize the word "Internet", it may surprise you to learn there is no "Internet, Inc.," no business in charge of this uniquely postmodern creation. Administration of this world-wide communication complex is still handled by the cooperating institutions and regional networks that comprise the Internet. The word "Internet" denotes a specific interconnected network of networks, and not a corporate entity.

Using the World Wide Web for Research

Just as no one owns the worldwide communication complex that is the Internet, there is no formal organization among the collection of hundreds of thousands of computers that make up the part of the Net called the World Wide Web.

If you've never seriously used the Web, you are about to take your first steps on what can only be described as an incredible journey. Initially, though, you might find it convenient to think of the Web as a giant television network with millions of channels. It's safe to say that, among all these channels, there's something for you to watch. Only, how to find it? You could click through the channels one by one, of course, but by the time you found something of interest it would (1) be over or (2) leave you wondering if there wasn't something better on that you're missing.

A more efficient way to search for what you want would be to consult some sort of TV listing. While you could skim through pages more rapidly than channels, the task would still be daunting. A more creative approach would allow you to press a button on your remote control that would connect you to a channel of interest; what's more, that channel would contain the names (or numbers) of other channels with similar programs. Those channels in turn would contain information about other channels. Now you could zip through this million-channel universe, touching down only at programs of potential interest. This seems far more effective than the hunt-and-peck method of the traditional couch potato.

If you have a feel for how this might work for television, you have a feel for what it's like to journey around (or surf) the Web. Instead of channels on the Web, we have *Web sites*. Each site contains one or more *pages*. Each page may contain, among other things, links to other pages, either in the same site or in other sites, anywhere in the world. These other pages may elaborate on the information you're looking at or may direct you to related but not identical information, or even provide contrasting or contradictory points of view; and, of course, these pages could have links of their own.

Web sites are maintained by businesses, institutions, affinity groups, professional organizations, government departments, and ordinary people anxious to express opinions, share information, sell products, or provide services. Because these Web sites are stored electronically, updating them is more convenient and practical than updating printed media. That makes Web sites far more dynamic than other types of research material you may be used to, and it means a visit to a Web site can open up new opportunities that weren't available as recently as a few hours ago.

part
1

Hypertext and Links

The invention that unveils these revolutionary possibilities is called *hypertext*. Hypertext is a technology for combining text, graphics, sounds, video, and links on a single World Wide Web page. Click on a link and you're transported, like Alice falling down the rabbit hole, to a new page, a new address, a new environment for research and communication.

Links come in three flavors: text, picture, and hot spot. A text link may be a letter, a word, a phrase, a sentence, or any contiguous combination of text characters. You can identify text links at a glance because

Text Link

Picture Link

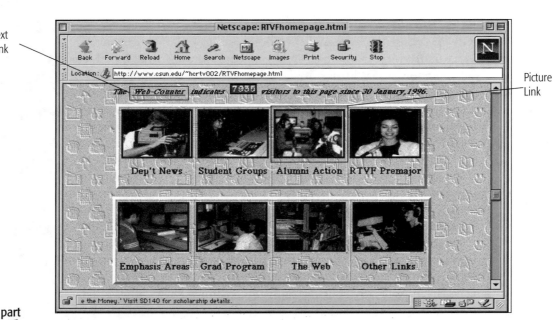

Text links are underlined and set of in color. Picture links are set off by a colored border. Hot spots carry no visual identification.

part

1

the characters are <u>underlined</u>, and are often displayed in a unique color, setting the link apart from the rest of the text on the page. Picture links are pictures or other graphic elements. On the Web, a picture may not only be worth a thousand words, but it may also be the start of a journey into a whole new corner of cyberspace.

The third kind of link, the hot spot, is neither underlined nor bordered, a combination which would make it impossible to spot, were it not for a Web convention that offers you a helping hand finding all types of links. This helping hand is, well, a hand. Whenever the mouse cursor passes over a link, the cursor changes from an arrow to a hand. Wherever you see the hand icon, you can click and retrieve another Web page. Sweep the cursor over an area of interest, see the hand, follow the link, and you're surfing the Web.

In the Name of the Page

Zipping around the Web in this way may seem exciting, even serendipitous, but it's also fraught with perils. How, for instance, do you revisit a page of particular interest? Or share a page with a classmate? Or cite a page as a reference for a professor? Web page designers assign names, or titles, to their pages; unfortunately, there's nothing to prevent two designers from assigning the same title to different pages.

An instrument that uniquely identifies Web pages does exist. It's called a Universal Resource Locator (URL), the cyber-signposts of the World Wide Web. URLs contain all the information necessary to locate:

- the page containing the information you're looking for;
- the computer that hosts (stores) that page of information;
- the form the information is stored in.

A typical URL looks like this:

```
http://www.abacon.com/homepage.html
```

You enter it into the **Location** field at the top of your browser window. Hit the **Return** (or **Enter**) key and your browser will deliver to your screen the exact page specified. When you click on a link, you're actually using a shorthand alternative to typing the URL yourself because the browser does it for you. In fact, if you watch the "Location" field when you click on a link, you'll see its contents change to the URL you're traveling to.

part
1

The URL Exposed

How does your browser—or the whole World Wide Web structure, for that matter—know where you're going? As arcane as the URL appears, there is a logical explanation to its apparent madness. (This is true not only of URLs but also of your computer experience in general. Because a computer's "intelligence" only extends to following simple instructions exactly, most of the commands, instructions, and procedures you'll encounter have simple underlying patterns. Once you familiarize yourself with these patterns, you'll find you're able to make major leaps in your understanding of new Internet features.)

To unscramble the mysteries of World Wide Web addresses, we'll start at the end of the URL and work our way toward the front.

```
/homepage.html
```

This is the name of a single file or document. Eventually, the contents of this file/document will be transferred over the Internet to your computer.

However, because there are undoubtedly thousands of files on the Internet with this name, we need to clarify our intentions a bit more.

`www.abacon.com`

This is the name of a particular Internet *Web server*, a computer whose job it is to forward Web pages to you on request. By Internet convention, this name is unique. The combination of

`www.abacon.com/homepage.html`

identifies a unique file/document on a unique Web server on the World Wide Web. No other file has this combined address, so there's no question about which file/document to transfer to you.

The characters *http://* at the beginning of the URL identify the method by which the file/document will be transferred. The letters stand for **H**yper**T**ext **T**ransfer **P**rotocol.

part

1

Quick Check

Don't Be Lost In (Hyper)Space

Let's pause for a quick check of your Web navigation skills. Look at the sample web page on the next page. How many links does it contain?

Did you find all five? That's right, five:

- The word "links" in the second line below the seaside picture;
- The sentence "What about me?";
- The word "cyberspace" in the quick brown fox sentence;
- The red and white graphic in the lower left-hand corner of the page. The blue border around it matches the blue of the text links;
- The hot spot in the seaside picture. We know there's at least one link in the picture, because the cursor appears as a hand. (There may be more hot spots on the page, but we can't tell from this picture alone.)

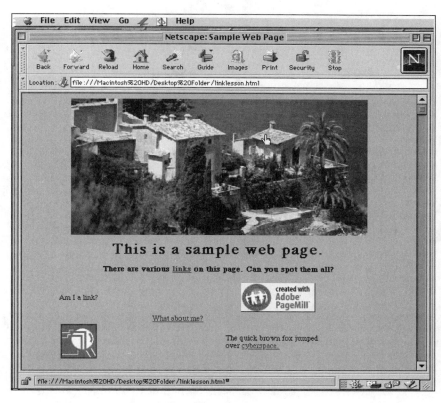

A sample web page to exercise your link identifying skills.

Getting There from Here

Now you know that a URL uniquely identifies a page and that links used as shorthand for URLs enable you to travel from page to page in the Web; but what if a link takes you someplace you don't want to go? Missing page messages take several forms, such as URL 404, Object not on this server, Missing Object, Page not Found, but they all lead to the same place—a dead end. The page specified by the link or URL no longer exists. There are many reasons for missing pages. You may have entered the URL incorrectly. Every character must be precise and no spaces are allowed. More than likely, though, especially if you arrived here via a link, the page you're after has been moved or removed. Remember, anybody can create a link to any page. In the spirit of the Internet, there are no forms to fill out, no procedures to follow. That's the

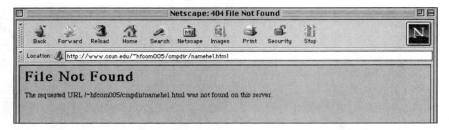

A missing page message, an all too common road hazard on the information superhighway.

good news. The bad news is that the owner of a page is under no obligation to inform the owners of links pointing to it that the page location has changed. In fact, there's no way for the page owner to even know about all the links to her page. Yes, the Internet's spirit of independence proves frustrating sometimes, but you'll find these small inconveniences are a cheap price to pay for the benefits you receive. Philosophy aside, though, we're still stuck on a page of no interest to us. The best strategy is to back up and try another approach.

Every time you click on the **Back** button, you return to the previous page you visited. That's because your browser keeps track of the pages you visit and the order in which you visit them. The **Back** icon, and its counterpart, the **Forward** icon, allow you to retrace the steps, forward and backward, of your cyberpath. Sometimes you may want to move two, three, or a dozen pages at once. Although you can click the **Back** or **Forward** icons multiple times, Web browsers offer an easier navigation shortcut. Clicking on the **Go** menu in the menu bar displays a list of your most recently visited pages, in the order you've been there. Unlike the **Back** or **Forward** icons, you can select any page from the menu, and a single click takes you directly there. There's no need to laboriously move one page at a time.

Quick Check

As a quick review, here's what we know about navigating the Web so far:

- Enter a URL directly into the Location field;
- Click on a link;
- Use the **Back** or **Forward** icons;
- Select a page from the **Go** menu.

You Can Go Home (and to Other Pages) Again

How do we return to a page hours, days, or even months later? One way is to write down the URLs of every page we may want to revisit. There's got to be a better way, and there is: We call them bookmarks (on Netscape Communicator) or favorites (on Microsoft Internet Explorer).

Like their print book namesakes, Web bookmarks (and favorites) flag specific Web pages. Selecting an item from the **Bookmark/Favorites** menu, like selecting an item from the **Go** menu, is the equivalent of entering a URL into the **Location** field of your browser, except that items in the **Bookmark/Favorites** menu are ones you've added yourself and represent pages visited over many surfing experiences, not just the most recent one.

To select a page from your bookmark list, pull down the **Bookmark/Favorites** menu and click on the desired entry. In Netscape Communicator, clicking on the **Add Bookmark** command makes a bookmark entry for the current page. **Add Page to Favorites** performs the same function in Microsoft Internet Explorer.

To save a favorite page location, use the **Add** feature available on both browsers. Clicking that feature adds the location of the current page to your **Bookmark/Favorites** menu. A cautionary note is in order here. Your bookmark or favorites list physically exists only on your personal computer, which means that if you connect to the Internet on a different computer, your list won't be available. If you routinely connect to the Internet from a computer lab, for example, get ready to carry the URLs for your favorite Web sites in your notebook or your head.

part

1

Searching and Search Engines

Returning to our cable television analogy, you may recall that we conveniently glossed over the question of how we selected a starting channel in the first place. With a million TV channels, or several million Web pages, we can't depend solely on luck guiding us to something interesting.

On the Web, we solve the problem with specialized computer programs called *search engines* that crawl through the Web, page by page, cataloging its contents. As different software designers developed search strategies, entrepreneurs established Web sites where any user could find pages containing particular words and phrases. Today, Web sites such as Yahoo!, AltaVista, Excite, WebCrawler, and MetaCrawler offer you a "front door" to the Internet that begins with a search for content of interest.

The URLs for some popular search sites are:

Excite	`www.excite.com`
Yahoo!	`www.yahoo.com`
AltaVista	`www.altavista.digital.com`
WebCrawler	`www.webcrawler.com`
MetaCrawler	`www.metacrawler.com`
Infoseek	`www.infoseek.com`
EBlast	`www.eblast.com`
HotBot	`www.hotbot.com`

Internet Gold Is Where You Find It

Let's perform a simple search using HotBot to find information about the history of the Internet.

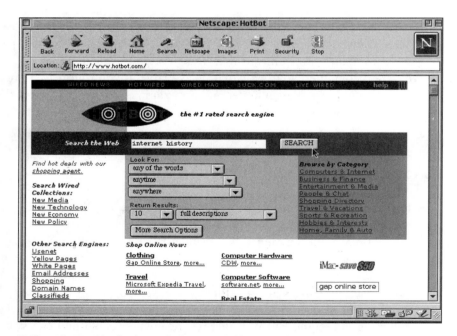

We'll start by searching for the words "internet" or "history." By looking for "any of the words," the search will return pages on which either "internet" or "history" or both appear.

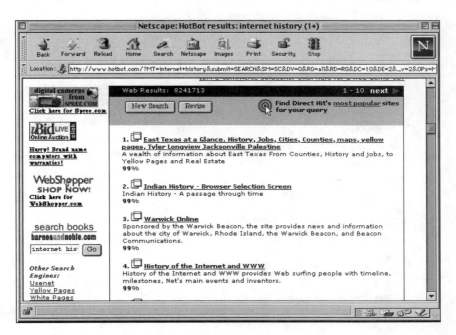

Our search returned 12,334,156 matches or *hits.* Note that the first two items don't seem to be Internet history–related. The percentage number in the last line of each summary indicates the "quality" of the match, usually related to the number of times the search word(s) appears on the page.

part

1

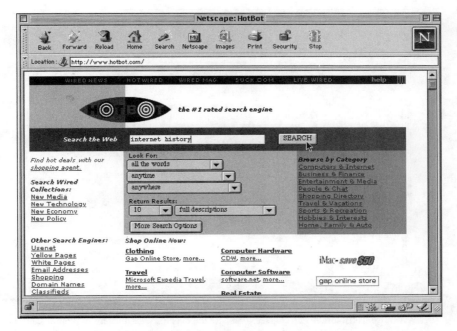

When we conduct the same search, but this time looking for "all the words," the search returns hits when both "internet" and "history" appear on the same page, in any order, and not necessarily next to each other.

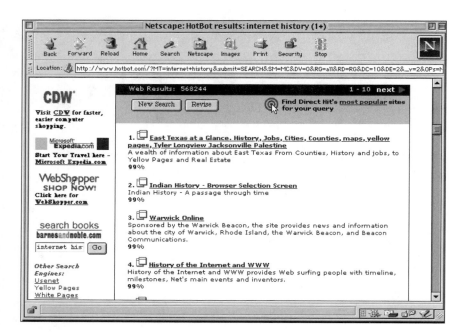

The search is narrowed down to only 885,911 hits. Note that the first four items are the same as in the previous search.

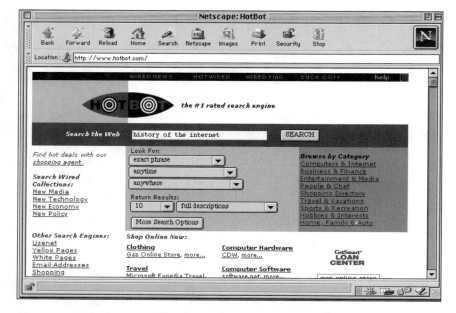

When we search for the exact phrase "history of the internet," which means those four words in exactly that order, with no intervening words, we're down to less than 12,000 hits (still a substantial number). This time, the first two hits look dead-on, and the third is a possibility, if we knew what "GTO" meant. The fourth hit is strange, so we click on it to check it out.

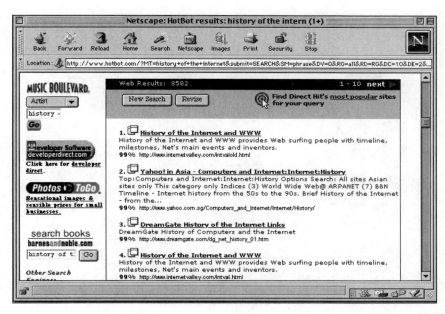

part

1

This hit seems to have nothing to do with the history of the Internet. Hits happen. No search engine is 100 percent accurate 100 percent of the time. Spurious search results are the serendipity of the Internet. Look at them as an opportunity to explore something new.

Out of curiosity, let's try our history of the Internet search using a different search engine. When we search for the phrase "history of the internet" using WebCrawler, the quotation marks serve the same purpose as selecting "the exact phrase" option in Hotbot. The WebCrawler search only finds 504 hits. Some are the same as those found using HotBot, some are different. Different searching strategies and software algorithms make using more than one search engine a must for serious researchers.

The major search engines conveniently provide you with tips to help you get the most out of their searches. These include ways to use AND and OR to narrow down searches, and ways to use NOT to eliminate unwanted hits.

Each search engine also uses a slightly different approach to cataloging the Web, so at different sites your results might vary. Often, one search engine provides better results (more relevant hits) in your areas of interest; sometimes, the wise strategy is to provide the same input to several different engines. No one search engine does a perfect job all the time, so experience will dictate the one that's most valuable for you.

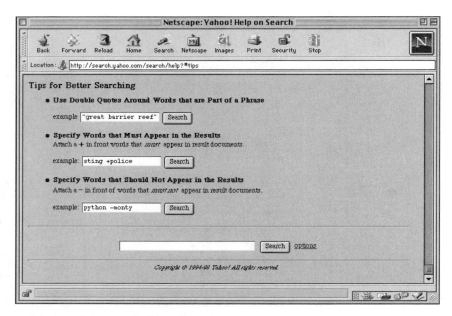

part

1

You'll find search tip pages like this at all the major searcch engine sites.

Quick Check

Let's review our searching strategies:

- ■ Visit one of the search engine sites;
- ■ Enter key words or phrases that best describe the search criteria;
- ■ Narrow the search if necessary by using options such as "all the words" or "the exact phrase." On some search engines, you may use the word "and" or the symbol "|" to indicate words that all must appear on a page;
- ■ Try using the same criteria with different search engines.

How Not to Come Down with a Virus

Downloading files from the Internet allows less responsible Net citizens to unleash onto your computer viruses, worms, and Trojan horses, all dangerous programs that fool you into thinking they're doing one thing while they're actually erasing your hard disk or performing some other undesirable task. Protection is your responsibility.

One way to reduce the risk of contracting a virus is to download software from reliable sites. Corporations such as Microsoft and Apple take care to make sure downloadable software is virus free. So do most institutions that provide software downloads as a public service (such as the Stanford University archives of Macintosh software). Be especially careful of programs you find on someone's home page. If you're not sure about safe download sources, ask around in a newsgroup (discussed shortly), talk to friends, or check with the information technology center on campus.

You can also buy and use a reliable virus program. Norton, Symantec, and Dr. Solomon all sell first-rate programs for the Mac and PC. You can update these programs right from the Internet so they'll detect the most current viruses. Most of the time, these programs can disinfect files/documents on your disk that contain viruses. Crude as it may sound, downloading programs from the Internet without using a virus check is like having unprotected sex with a stranger. While downloading software may not be life threatening, imagine the consequences if your entire hard disk, including all your course work and software, is totally obliterated. It won't leave you feeling very good.

part
1

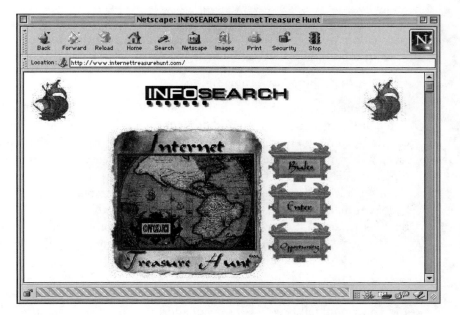

If you'd like some entertaining practice sharpening your Web searching skills, point your browser to <www.internettreasurehunt.com>, follow the directions, and you're on your way to becoming an Internet researcher extraordinaire.

The (E)mail Goes Through

Email was one of the first applications created for the Internet by its designers, who sought a method of communicating with each other directly from their keyboards. Your electronic Internet mailbox is to email what a post office box is to "snail mail" (the name Net citizens apply to ordinary, hand-delivered mail). This mailbox resides on the computer of your Internet Service Provider (ISP). That's the organization providing you with your Internet account. Most of the time your ISP will be your school; but, you may contract with one of the commercial providers, such as America Online, Netcom, Microsoft Network, Earthlink, or AT&T. The Internet doesn't deliver a message to your door but instead leaves it in a conveniently accessible place (your mailbox) in the post office (the computer of your ISP), until you retrieve the mail using your combination (password).

If you currently have computer access to the Internet, your school or ISP assigned you a *user name* (also called a user id, account name, or account number). This user name may be your first name, your first initial and the first few characters of your last name, or some strange combination of numbers and letters only a computer could love. An email address is a combination of your user name and the unique address of the computer through which you access your email, like this:

    username@computername.edu

The three letters after the dot, in this case "edu," identify the top level "domain." There are six common domain categories in use: edu (educational), com (commercial), org (organization), net (network), mil (military), and gov (government). The symbol "@"—called the "at" sign in typewriter days—serves two purposes: For computers, it provides a neat, clean separation between your user name and the computer name; for people, it makes Internet addresses more pronounceable. Your address is read: user name "at" computer name "dot" e-d-u. Suppose your Internet user name is "a4736g" and your ISP is Allyn & Bacon, the publisher of this book. Your email address might look like

    a4736g@abacon.com

and you would tell people your email address is "ay-four-seven-three-six-gee at ay bacon dot com."

We Don't Just Handle Your Email, We're Also a Client

You use email with the aid of special programs called *mail clients*. As with search engines, mail clients have the same set of core features, but your access to these features varies with the type of program. On both the PC and the Mac, Netscape Communicator and Microsoft Internet Explorer give you access to mail clients while you're plugged into the Web. That way you can pick up and send mail while you're surfing the Web.

The basic email service functions are creating and sending mail, reading mail, replying to mail, and forwarding mail. First we'll examine the process of sending and reading mail, and then we'll discuss how to set up your programs so that your messages arrive safely.

Let's look at a typical mail client screen, in this case from Netscape Communicator 4. You reach this screen by choosing **Messenger Inbox** from the menu. Along the top of the screen are icons denoting the basic mail service functions. To send a message from scratch, choose the **New Msg** icon to create a blank message form, which has fields for the recipient's address and the subject, and a window for the text of the message.

Fill in the recipient's address in the "To" field, just above the arrow. Use your own address. We'll send email to ourselves and use the same

part

1

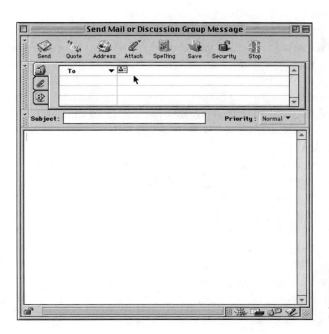

New message form, with fields for recipient's address and the subject, and a window for the text of the message.

message to practice sending email and reading it as well; then we'll know if your messages come out as expected.

Click in the "Subject" field and enter a word or phrase that generally describes the topic of the message. Since we're doing this for the first time, let's type "Maiden Email Voyage."

Now click anywhere in the text window and enter your message. Let's say "Hi. Thanks for guiding me through sending my first email." You'll find that the mail client works here like a word processing program, which means you can insert and delete words and characters and highlight text.

Now click the **Send** icon. You've just created and sent your first email message. In most systems, it takes a few seconds to a few minutes for a message to yourself to reach your mailbox, so you might want to take a short break before continuing. When you're ready to proceed, close the **Send Mail** window and click the **Get Msg** icon in the **Inbox** window.

What Goes Around Comes Around

Now let's grab hold of the message you just sent to yourself. When retrieving mail, most mail clients display a window showing the messages in your mailbox telling you how many new messages have been added.

If you've never used your email before, chances are your message window is empty, or contains only one or two messages (usually official messages from the ISP) besides the one you sent to yourself. The message to yourself should be accompanied by an indicator of some sort—a colored mark, the letter N—indicating it's a new message. In Netscape Communicator, as in other mail clients, you also get to see the date of the message, who sent it, and the information you entered in the subject line. The Subject field lets you scan your messages and determine which ones you want to look at first.

The summary of received messages tells you everything you need to know about a message except what's in it. Click anywhere in the line to see the contents in the message window. Click on the message from yourself and you'll see the contents of the message displayed in a window. The information at the top—To, From, Subject, and so forth—is called the *header*. Depending on your system, you may also see some cryptic lines with terms such as X-Mailer, received by, and id number. Most of the time, there's nothing in this part of the header of interest, so just skip over it for now.

Moving Forward

The contents, or text, of your message can be cut and pasted just like any other text document. If you and a classmate are working on a project together, your partner can write part of a paper and email it to you, and you can copy the text from your email message and paste it into your word processing program.

What if there are three partners in this project? One partner sends you a draft of the paper for you to review. You like it and want to send it on to your other partner. The **Forward** feature lets you send the message intact, so you don't have to cut and paste it into a new message window. To forward a message, highlight it in the **Inbox** (top) and click the **Forward** icon. Enter the recipient's address in the "To" field of the message window. Note that the subject of the message is "Fwd:" followed by the subject of the original message. Use the text window to add your comments ahead of the original message.

A Chance to Reply

part **1**

Email is not a one-way message system. Let's walk through a reply to a message from a correspondent named Elliot. Highlight the message in your **Inbox** again and this time click on the **Reply** icon. When the message window appears, click on the **Quote** icon. Depending on which program you're using, you'll see that each line in the message is preceded by either a vertical bar or a right angle bracket (>).

Note the vertical line to the left of the original text. The "To" and "Subject" fields are filled in automatically with the address of the sender and the original subject preceded by "Re:". In Internet terminology, the message has been *quoted*. The vertical bar or > is used to indicate lines not written by you but by someone else (in this case, the message's original author). Why bother? Because this feature allows you to reply without retyping the parts of the message you're responding to. Because your typing isn't quoted, your answers stand out from the original message. Netscape Communicator 4 adds some blank lines above and below your comments, a good practice for you if your mail client doesn't do this automatically.

Welcome to the Internet, Miss Manners

While we're on the subject of email, here are some *netiquette* (net etiquette) tips.

- When you send email to someone, even someone who knows you well, all they have to look at are your words—there's no body language attached. That means there's no smile, no twinkle in the eye, no raised eyebrow; and especially, there's no tone of voice. What you write is open to interpretation and your recipient has nothing to guide him or her. You may understand the context of a remark, but will your reader? If you have any doubts about how your message will be interpreted, you might want to tack on an *emoticon* to your message. An emoticon is a face created out of keyboard characters. For example, there's the happy Smiley :-) (you have to look at it sideways . . . the parenthesis is its mouth), the frowning Smiley :-((Frownie?), the winking Smiley ;-), and so forth. Smileys are the body language of the Internet. Use them to put remarks in context. "Great," in response to a friend's suggestion means you like the idea. "Great :-(" changes the meaning to one of disappointment or sarcasm. (Want a complete list of emoticons? Try using "emoticon" as a key word for a Web search.)

- Keep email messages on target. One of the benefits of email is its speed. Reading through lengthy messages leaves the reader wondering when you'll get to the point.

- Email's speed carries with it a certain responsibility. Its ease of use and the way a messages seems to cry out for an answer both encourage quick responses, but quick doesn't necessarily mean thoughtful. Once you hit the **Send** icon, that message is gone. There's no recall button. Think before you write, lest you feel the wrath of the modern-day version of your parents' adage: Answer in haste, repent at leisure.

Keeping Things to Yourself

Here's another tip cum cautionary note, this one about Web security. Just as you take care to protect your wallet or purse while walking down a crowded street, it's only good practice to exercise caution with information you'd like to keep (relatively) private. Information you pass around the Internet is stored on, or passed along by, computers that are accessible to others. Although computer system administrators take great care to insure the security of this information, no scheme is completely infallible. Here are some security tips:

part
1

■ Exercise care when sending sensitive information such as credit card numbers, passwords, even telephone numbers and addresses in plain email. Your email message may pass through four or five computers en route to its destination, and at any of these points, it can be intercepted and read by someone other than the recipient.

■ Send personal information over the Web only if the page is secure. Web browsers automatically encrypt information on secure pages, and the information can only be unscrambled at the Web site that created the secure page. You can tell if a page is secure by checking the status bar at the bottom of your browser's window for an icon of a closed lock.

■ Remember that any files you store on your ISP's computer are accessible to unscrupulous hackers.

■ Protect your password. Many Web client programs, such as mail clients, have your password for you. That means anyone with physical access to your computer can read your email. With a few simple tools, someone can even steal your password. Never leave your password on a lab computer. (Make sure the **Remember Password** or **Save Password** box is unchecked in any application that asks for your password.)

part
1

The closed lock icon in the lower left-hand corner of your browser window indicates a "secure" Web page.

An Audience Far Wider Than You Imagine

Remember that the Web in particular and the Internet in general are communications mediums with a far-reaching audience, and placing information on the Internet is tantamount to publishing it. Certainly, the contents of any message or page you post become public information, but in a newsgroup (an electronic bulletin board), your email address also becomes public knowledge. On a Web page, posting a photo of your favorite music group can violate the photographer's copyright, just as if you published the image in a magazine. Use common sense about posting information you or someone else expects to remain private; and, remember, information on the Web can and will be read by people with different tastes and sensitivities. The Web tends to be self-censoring, so be prepared to handle feedback, both good and bad.

A Discussion of Lists

There's no reason you can't use email to create a discussion group. You pose a question, for example, by sending an email message to everyone in the group. Somebody answers and sends the answer to everyone else on the list, and so on.

At least, that's the theory.

In practice, this is what often happens. As people join and leave the group, you and the rest of your group are consumed with updating your lists, adding new names and deleting old ones. As new people join, their addresses may not make it onto the lists of all the members of the group, so different participants get different messages. The work of administering the lists becomes worse than any value anyone can get out of the group, and so it quickly dissolves.

Generally, you're better off letting the computer handle discussion group administration. A *list server* is a program for administering emailing lists. It automatically adds and deletes list members and handles the distribution of messages.

part
1

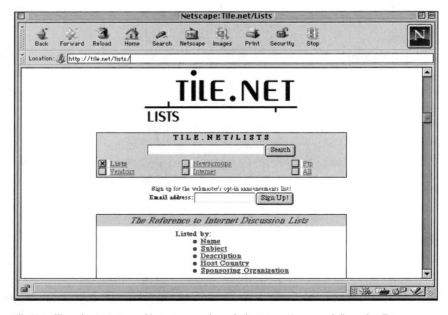

Tile.Net offfers shortcuts to working your way through the Internet's maze of discussion lists.

Thousands of mailing lists have already been formed by users with common interests. You may find mailing lists for celebrities, organizations, political interests, occupations, and hobbies. Your instructor may establish a mailing list for your course.

Groups come in several different flavors. Some are extremely active. You can receive as many as forty or more email messages a day. Other lists may send you a message a month. One-way lists, such as printed newsletters, do not distribute your reply to any other subscriber. Some lists distribute replies to everyone. These lists include mediated lists, in which an "editor" reviews each reply for suitability (relevance, tone, use of language) before distributing the message, and unmediated lists, in which each subscriber's response is automatically distributed to all the other subscribers with no restrictions except those dictated by decency and common sense, though these qualities may not always be obvious from reading the messages.

Get on a List Online

You join in the discussion by subscribing to a list, which is as straightforward as sending email. You need to know only two items: the name of the list and the address of the list server program handling subscriptions. To join a list, send a **Subscribe** message to the list server address. The message must contain the letters "Sub," the name of the list, and your name (your real name, not your user name), all on one line. *And that's all.* This message will be read by a computer program that looks for these items only. At the very best, other comments in the message will be ignored. At the very worst, your entire message will be ignored, and so will you.

Within a few hours to a day after subscribing, the list server will automatically send you a confirmation email message, including instructions for sending messages, finding out information about the list and its members, and canceling your subscription. Save this message for future reference. That way, if you do decide to leave the list, you won't have to circulate a message to the members asking how to unsubscribe, and you won't have to wade through fifty replies all relaying the same information you received when you joined.

Soon after your confirmation message appears in your mailbox, and depending on the activity level of the list, you'll begin receiving email messages. New list subscribers customarily wait a while before joining the discussion. After all, you're electronically strolling into a room full of strangers; it's only fair to see what topics are being discussed before

part

1

wading in with your own opinions. Otherwise, you're like the bore at the party who elbows his way into a conversation with "But enough about you, let's talk about me." You'll also want to avoid the faux pas of posting a long missive on a topic that subscribers spent the preceding three weeks thrashing out. Observe the list for a while, understand its tone and feel, what topics are of interest to others and what areas are taboo. Also, look for personalities. Who's the most vociferous? Who writes very little but responds thoughtfully? Who's the most flexible? The most rigid? Most of all, keep in mind that there are far more observers than participants. What you write may be read by 10 or 100 times more people than those whose names show up in the daily messages.

When you reply to a message, you reply to the list server address, not to the address of the sender (unless you intend for your communication to remain private). The list server program takes care of distributing your message listwide. Use the address in the "Reply To" field of the message. Most mail clients automatically use this address when you select the **Reply** command. Some may ask if you want to use the reply address (say yes). Some lists will send a copy of your reply to you so you know your message is online. Others don't send the author a copy, relying on your faith in the infallibility of computers.

In the words of those famous late night television commercials, you can cancel your subscription at any time. Simply send a message to the address you used to subscribe (which you'll find on that confirmation message you saved for reference), with "Unsub," followed on the same line by the name of the list. For example, to leave a list named "WRITER-L," you would send:

```
Unsub WRITER-L
```

Even if you receive messages for a short while afterwards, have faith—they will disappear.

Waste Not, Want Not

List servers create an excellent forum for people with common interests to share their views; however, from the Internet standpoint, these lists are terribly wasteful. First of all, if there are one thousand subscribers to a list, every message must be copied one thousand times and distributed over the Internet. If there are forty replies a day, this one list creates forty thousand email messages. Ten such lists mean almost a half million messages, most of which are identical, flying around the Net.

Another wasteful aspect of list servers is the way in which messages are answered. The messages in your mailbox on any given day represent a combination of new topics and responses to previous messages. But where are these previous messages? If you saved them, they're in your email mailbox taking up disk space. If you haven't saved them, you have nothing to compare the response to. What if a particular message touches off a chain of responses, with subscribers referring not only to the source message but to responses as well? It sounds like the only safe strategy is to save every message from the list, a suggestion as absurd as it is impractical.

What we really need is something closer to a bulletin board than a mailing list. On a bulletin board, messages are posted once. Similar notices wind up clustered together. Everyone comes to the same place to read or post messages.

And Now the News(group)

part
1

The Internet equivalent of the bulletin board is the Usenet or newsgroup area. Usenet messages are copied only once for each ISP supporting the newsgroup. If there are one thousand students on your campus reading the same newsgroup message, there need only be one copy of the message stored on your school's computer.

Categorizing a World of Information

Newsgroups are categorized by topics, with topics broken down into subtopics and sub-subtopics. For example, you'll find newsgroups devoted to computers, hobbies, science, social issues, and "alternatives." Newsgroups in this last category cover a wide range of topics that may not appeal to the mainstream. Also in this category are beginning newsgroups.

Usenet names are amalgams of their topics and subtopics, separated by dots. If you were interested in a newsgroup dealing with, say, music, you might start with rec.music and move down to rec.music.radiohead, or rec.music.techno, and so forth. The naming scheme allows you to zero in on a topic of interest.

Getting into the News(group) Business

Most of the work of reading, responding to, and posting messages is handled by a news reader client program, accessible through both Netscape Communicator and Microsoft Internet Explorer. You can not only surf the Web and handle your mail via your browser, but you can also drop into your favorite newsgroups virtually all in one operation.

Let's drop into a newsgroup. To reach groups via Netscape Communicator, select the **Message Center** icon, then select "news" from the message center window. Your news reader displays a list of available groups. In Netscape Communicator, this list appears in outline form to save space. Click on the arrows next to the folder names to move down the outline (through the categories) to see more groups.

To subscribe to a newsgroup—that is, to tell your news reader you want to be kept up-to-date on the messages posted to a particular group—highlight the group of interest and click on **Subscribe.** Alternately, you can click in the Subscribe column to the right of the group name. The check mark in the Subscribe column means you're "in."

The message center in Netscape Communicator displays a list of newsgroups on your subscription list. Double click on the one of current interest and your reader presents you with a list of messages posted on the group's bulletin board. Double click on a message to open its contents in a window.

Often, messages contain "Re:" in their subject lines, indicating a response to a previous message (the letters stand for "Regarding"). Many news readers maintain a *thread* for you. Threads are chains of messages and all responses to that message. These readers give you the option to read messages chronologically or to read a message followed by its responses.

When you subscribe to a newsgroup, your news reader will also keep track of the messages you've read so that it can present you with the newest (unread) ones. While older messages are still available to you, this feature guarantees that you stay up-to-date without any record keeping on your part. Subscribing to a newsgroup is free, and the subscription information resides on your computer.

Newsgroups have no way of knowing who their subscribers are, and the same caveat that applies to bookmarks applies to newsgroups. Information about your subscriptions resides physically on the personal computer you're using. If you switch computers, as in a lab, your subscription information and history of read messages are beyond your reach.

part

1

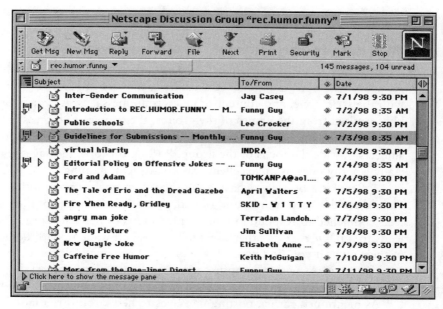

A listing of posted messages. While not visible from this black and white reproduction, a red indicator in the Subject column marks unread messages.

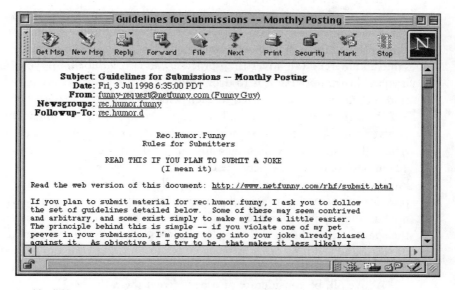

Double-clicking on a message opens its contents into a window like this. You can reply to this message via the Reply icon, or get the next message using the Next icon.

Welcome to the Internet, Miss Manners—Again

As with list servers, hang out for a while, or *lurk*, to familiarize yourself with the style, tone, and content of newsgroup messages. As you probably surmised from the names of the groups, their topics of discussion are quite narrow. One of the no-nos of newsgroups is posting messages on subjects outside the focus of the group. Posting off-topic messages, especially lengthy ones, is an excellent way to attract a flaming.

A *flame* is a brutally debasing message from one user to another. Flames are designed to hurt and offend, and often the target of the flame feels compelled to respond in kind to protect his or her self-esteem. This leads to a *flame war,* as other users take sides and wade in with flames of their own. If you find yourself the target of a flame, your best strategy is to ignore it. As with a campfire, if no one tends to the flames, they soon die out.

As mentioned earlier, posting messages to newsgroups is a modern form of publishing, and a publisher assumes certain responsibilities. You have a duty to keep your messages short and to the point. Many newsgroup visitors connect to the Internet via modems. Downloading a day's worth of long postings, especially uninteresting ones, is annoying and frustrating. Similarly, don't post the same message to multiple, related newsgroups. This is called *cross posting,* and it's a peeve of Net citizens who check into these groups. If you've ever flipped the television from channel to channel during a commercial break only to encounter the same commercial (an advertising practice called *roadblocking*), you can imagine how annoying it is to drop in on several newsgroups only to find the same messages posted to each one.

With the huge potential audience newsgroups offer, you might think you've found an excellent medium for advertising goods or services. After all, posting a few messages appears analogous to running classified ads in newspapers, only here the cost is free. There's a name for these kinds of messages—*spam.* Spam is the junk mail of the Internet, and the practice of spamming is a surefire way to attract flames. The best advice for handling spam? Don't answer it. Not only does an answer encourage the spammer, but he or she will also undoubtedly put your email address on a list and sell it to other spammers, who will flood your online mailbox with their junk.

Above all, be considerate of others. Treat them the way you'd like to be treated. Do you enjoy having your grammar or word choices corrected in front of the whole world? Do you feel comfortable when someone calls you stupid in public? Do you appreciate having your religion, ethnicity, heritage, or gender belittled in front of an audience? Respect the rights and feelings of others, if not out of simple decency then out of the sanctions your ISP may impose. Although you have every right to express an unpopular opinion or to take issue with the postings of others, most ISPs have regulations about the kinds of messages one can send via their facilities. Obscenities, threats, and spam may, at a minimum, result in your losing your Internet access privileges.

Give Your Web Browser Some Personality—Yours

Before accessing email and newsgroup functions, you need to set up or personalize your browser. If you always work on the same personal computer, this is a one-time operation that takes only a few minutes. In it, you tell your browser where to find essential computer servers, along with personal information the Internet needs to move messages for you.

part

1

- *Step 1:* Open the **Preferences** menu. In Netscape Communicator, it's located under the **Edit** menu; in Microsoft Internet Explorer, it's among the icons at the top of the screen.

- *Step 2:* Tell the browser who you are and where to find your mail servers. Your Reply To address is typically the same as your email address, though if you have an email alias you can use it here. Microsoft Internet Explorer has slots for your mail servers in the same window. Your ISP will provide the server names and addresses. Be sure to use your user name (and not your alias) in the "Account Name" field. SMTP handles your outgoing messages, while the POP3 server routes incoming mail. Often, but not always, these server names are the same. Netscape Communicator has a separate window for server names.

- *Step 3:* Tell the browser where to find your news server. Your ISP will furnish the name of the server. Note that in Microsoft Internet Explorer, you specify a helper application to read the news. Now that most computers come with browsers already loaded onto the hard disk, you'll find that these helper applications are already set up for you.

- *Step 4:* Set your home page. For convenience, you may want your browser to start by fetching a particular page, such as your favorite search site. Or you might want to begin at your school library's home page. Enter the URL for this starting page in the home page address field. Both Netscape and Microsoft offer the option of no home page when you start up. In that case, you get a blank browser window.

Operating systems such as Mac OS 8 and Microsoft Windows 95 offer automated help in setting up your browsers for Web, mail, and newsgroup operation. You need to know the names of the servers mentioned above, along with your user name and other details, such as the address of the domain name server (DNS) of your ISP. You should receive all this information when you open your Internet account. If not, ask for it.

Health Information on the Internet

part

1

Information relating to health, wellness, health care, and medicine abounds on the Internet. Web sites relating to any aspect of health are available with a few mouse clicks. What formerly took hours of searching for information from libraries can now be found in minutes. In former times, contacting colleagues to discuss important ideas required either a long distance phone call or a letter. Now, the Internet allows easy and immediate transmission of these ideas. Like-minded people from all over the world can now discuss ideas, pose questions, and receive new information at lightning speed—literally. The Internet has allowed health information to move to a new and very exciting level of distribution.

With the arrival of the Internet, people looking for health information can find it at every level. For the second grader who wants to learn about the differences between a fruit and a vegetable, it takes little time to find appropriate Web sites to gather this information. For the high school student who needs to write a report on the global situation of HIV and AIDS, information is readily available on the Internet. Similarly, for the scholarly researcher who is looking for information to support a theory on which to build a research study, the avenues are available on the Internet to find this type of information. The Internet has information relevant to every level of learning and there is almost no end to the quantity as well.

One of the premier locations for finding any type of health related information on the Internet is at a Web site called "Your Business, Your Health." This site can help you access nearly any type of health information that is online. This includes health news, health research, online health journals and magazines, and locations for doing health research. It also is an excellent starting place for finding information-specific health topics. The address for this Web site is: http://www.siu.edu/departments/bushea/

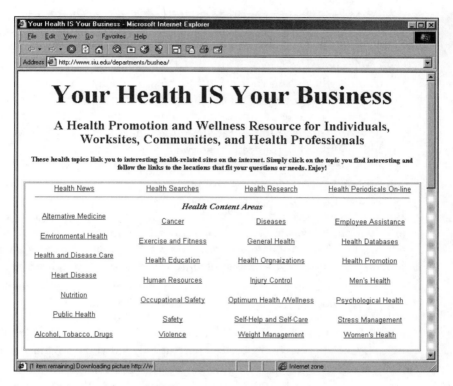

http://www.siu.edu/departments/bushea/

Using the Internet for Health Communication, Education, and Research

The Internet has quickly turned into an ocean of information for anyone who wants to know more about any aspect of health. A quick peek at any search engine (a Web site that allows you to search for something on the Internet) such as Yahoo! or AltaVista will quickly give us an idea of its immense size. For example, if we point our browser in the direction

part

1

of the Lycos A2Z search and then click on the words "Health and Medicine" we immediately move to a page that lists the following topics: Alternative Medicine, Death & Dying, Dentistry, Disabilities, Environmental Medicine, Ethics & Legal Issues in Health, Family Medical Almanac, Family Medicine, Hospitals & Clinics, Human Sexuality, Illnesses & Disorders, Medical History, Medical Insurance, Medical Research, Mental Health, Nutrition & Wellness, Occupational Medicine, Parenting, Pharmaceuticals, Professional Medicine, Public Health, and Public Policy Issues relating to health. Clicking on any of these topic areas will take us to long lists of related Web sites.

You may be asking yourself, "If there is so much information out there, where does a person begin when researching a subject or just wanting to know one particular idea?" For example, you may just want to know how many grams of fat are in the dinner you just ate at McDonald's. With a little bit of patience and following the steps and Internet addresses found in this book, you will be surprised how quickly you can find that for which you are looking.

part

1

Health topics on the information highway come from many different avenues. Many Web sites are designed for the sole purpose of giving out information. For example, a Web page dealing with weight control may tell you little more than data on foods and the various nutrients that are found in the foods. Other, more elaborate Web sites on weight control may have you fill out a questionnaire and then, based on your individual information, give you a printout of such information that is a bit more tailored to your needs. For example, it might let you know about the number of calories you need to consume daily to maintain, lose or gain weight. Considering your questionnaire, it may tell you how much exercise you ought to do during a typical week. It may give you pointers about what to look for on a food label to keep your intake of fats and sugars at a desirable level. Some Web sites are more interactive than others. The quality of the health related Web sites are as varied as the content.

Another aspect of the Internet, which makes it quite appealing to those looking for health information, is the global nature of the Internet. People from all parts of the world can contribute to this sea of information as easily as can someone from North Carolina or Oregon. The rich diversity of the Internet brings some unique and interesting answers to many health questions. What makes this even more interesting is that many times, those who create these very interesting and unique Web pages place their email address somewhere on the page so you can immediately and easily contact them. Suppose you were reading someone's page on some type of alternative medicine for which you previously had no understanding. Perhaps after completing this information you still had some questions. Using the Internet and email you can easily set up a dialogue with that person by sending them a letter and asking them your specific questions.

Never before has it been so simple to learn all you could ever want to know on just about any topic relating to health. At times it can be frustrating when you consider the enormous number of choices. With some patience and practice, however, you are certainly going to enjoy the effectiveness and usefulness of the Internet at whatever level of researching you might find yourself.

Locating Addresses for Health Professionals

One of the amazing things of the Internet is the instant ability to find people and send letters to them. A perfect example of this occurs with health professionals. Imagine that you went to a health conference or watched television and you heard someone speak on a topic that very much interested you. After the conference was over, you wanted to contact that person to ask some questions that were not asked in the meeting. Using the Internet, you can quickly find the email address to that person and write him or her a letter. Finding someone's email address is not very difficult. To begin with, there are search engines that find email addresses (mentioned earlier). Additionally, many health educators and health professionals have their email addresses listed at specific locations. One of these places to find email addresses for health educators is located at: http://131.230.221.136/hedir

Simply click on one of the directories listed by job site, by name, or by state and country, and you will find the names of many health education professionals around the world.

Locating a Newsgroup

Another way of gathering great health information is by connecting with a newsgroup. A newsgroup exists for nearly every aspect of health that you could imagine. About the only way to learn if a health related news-

part
1

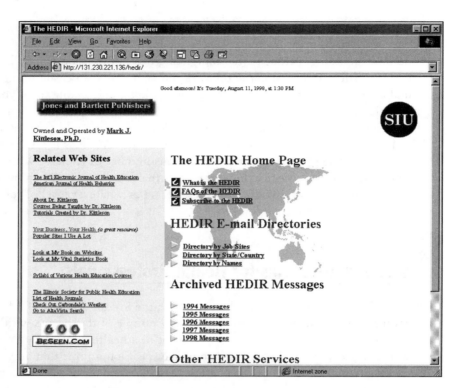

`http://131.230.221.136/hedir`

group might be interesting to you would be to check it out for yourself. Finding these newsgroups is not too difficult. You may type the words "health newsgroups" in your favorite search engine and see what you discover. After entering your request, the search engine will bring up many pages that list these health related newsgroups. One such page is titled "Health A2Z: The Search Engine for Health & Medicine." Its newsgroups URL (Internet address) is: http://www.healthatoz.com/categories/NG.htm

A long list of health related newsgroups appears. You may choose from any one of these that look particularly interesting. The titles in the listing usually give you an idea of the focus for each newsgroup. Some of the newsgroups to choose from at this point include the following: alt.hypnosis, alt.meditation, misc.fitness, misc.health.alternative, misc.health.diabetes, misc.kids.health, rec.food.veg, sci.life-extension, sci.med.aids, sci.med.diseases.cancer, sci.med.nutrition, and talk.politics.medicine to name a few.

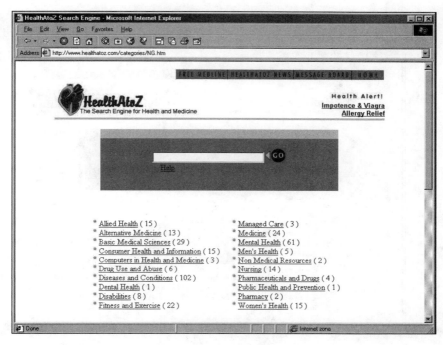

http://www.healthatoz.com/categories/NG.htm

part 1

Finding a Health Mailing List

There are certainly no shortage of mail lists for health. If you have never participated in a mailing list, doing so can seem intimidating. "Health A2Z: Mailing lists" (http://www.healthatoz.com/categories/ML.htm) is one of the best "first stops" to locate a health mailing list that you may find interesting. It includes an enormous directory of mailing lists including such topic areas as: Allied Health, Consumer Health, Drug Use and Abuse, Diseases and Conditions, Fitness and Exercise, Men's Health, Women's Health, and Public Health & Prevention to name only a few. Once you arrive at this first page, simply click on one of the topics, follow the instructions, and very soon you are part of a mailing list.

Some mailing lists have several thousand people who read and contribute to the lists. With that many people, the possibility of a very large number of daily letters in your mailbox is high. At first it might seem exciting to receive that much email. If you subscribe to more than

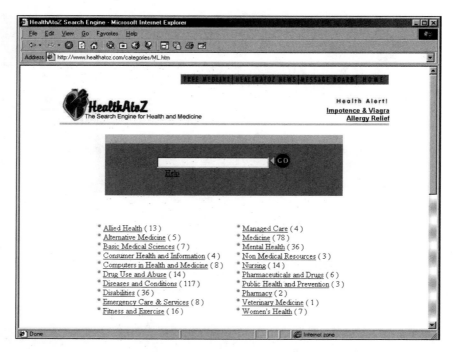

http://www.healthatoz.com/categories/ML.htm

one of these mailing lists, you will be receiving an even larger number of email letters each day. It is wise to determine the amount of time you have to read your email. Follow the feel of the list for a month or two and see if you want to remain subscribed to that list. Additionally, to avoid filling your mailbox, it is useful to set your browser to check your mailbox from time to time. Usually one check every hour or two is sufficient.

A Word to the Wise . . .

No longer is it a struggle to find what you need using the Internet. Be sure, however, to remember that there is no regulation as to what is produced on the Web. You do not have any way of determining the accuracy of information, so be careful. If you find information that is questionable or does not sound right, search elsewhere to get a second and third opinion. Use common sense when you are searching. If you are unsure about where to begin your search, refer to the Web sites in this manual as a guide. Happy surfing!

Critical Evaluation

Where Seeing Is Not Always Believing

Typical research resources, such as journal articles, books, and other scholarly works, are reviewed by a panel of experts before being published. At the very least, any reputable publisher takes care to assure that the author is who he or she claims to be and that the work being published represents a reasoned and informed point of view. When anyone can post anything in a Web site or to a newsgroup, the burden of assessing the relevance and accuracy of what you read falls to you. Rumors quickly grow into facts on the Internet simply because stories can spread so rapidly that the "news" seems to be everywhere. Because the Internet leaves few tracks, in no time it's impossible to tell whether you are reading independent stories or the merely same story that's been around the world two or three times. Gathering information on the Internet may be quick, but verifying the quality of information requires a serious commitment.

part

1

    Approach researching via the Internet with confidence, however, and not with trepidation. You'll find it an excellent workout for your critical evaluation skills; no matter what career you pursue, employers value an employee who can think critically and independently. Critical thinking is also the basis of problem solving, another ability highly valued by the business community. So, as you research your academic projects, be assured that you're simultaneously developing lifelong expertise.

It's Okay to Be Critical of Others

The first tip for successful researching on the Internet is to always consider your source. A Web site's URL often alerts you to the sponsor of the site. CNN or MSNBC are established news organizations, and you can give the information you find at their sites the same weight you would give to their cablecasts. Likewise, major newspapers operate Web sites with articles reprinted from their daily editions or expanded stories written expressly for the Internet. On the other hand, if you're unfamiliar with the source, treat the information the way you would any new data. Look for specifics—"66 percent of all voters" as opposed to "most voters"—and for information that can be verified—a cited report in another medium or information accessible through a Web site hosted by a credible sponsor—as opposed to generalities or unverifiable claims. Look for independent paths to the same information. This can involve careful use of search engines or visits to newsgroups with both similar and opposing viewpoints. Make sure that the "independent" information you find is truly independent. In newsgroups don't discount the possibility of multiple postings, or that a posting in one group is nothing more than a quotation from a posting in another. Ways to verify independent paths include following sources (if any) back to their origins, contacting the person posting a message and asking for clarification, or checking other media for verification.

In many cases, you can use your intuition and common sense to raise your comfort level about the soundness of the information. With both list servers and newsgroups, it's possible to lurk for a while to develop a feeling for the authors of various postings. Who seems the most authoritarian, and who seems to be "speaking" from emotion or bias? Who seems to know what he or she is talking about on a regular basis? Do these people cite their sources of information (a job or affiliation perhaps)? Do they have a history of thoughtful, insightful postings, or do their postings typically contain generalities, unjustifiable claims, or flames? On Web sites, where the information feels more anonymous, there are also clues you can use to test for authenticity. Verify who's hosting the Web site. If the host or domain name is unfamiliar to you, perhaps a search engine can help you locate more information. Measure the tone and style of the writing at the site. Does it seem consistent with the education level and knowledge base necessary to write intelligently about the subject?

When offering an unorthodox point of view, good authors supply facts, figures, and quotes to buttress their positions, expecting readers to be skeptical of their claims. Knowledgeable authors on the Internet follow these same commonsense guidelines. Be suspicious of authors who expect you to agree with their points of view simply because they've published them on the Internet. In one-on-one encounters, you frequently judge the authority and knowledge of the speaker using criteria you'd be hard pressed to explain. Use your sense of intuition on the Internet, too.

As a researcher (and as a human being), the job of critical thinking requires a combination of healthy skepticism and rabid curiosity. Newsgroups and Web sites tend to focus narrowly on single issues (newsgroups more so than Web sites). Don't expect to find a torrent of opposing views on newsgroup postings; their very nature and reason for existence dampens free-ranging discussions. A newsgroup on *The X-Files* might argue about whether extraterrestrials exist but not whether the program is the premier television show on the air today. Such a discussion

part

1

would run counter to the purposes of the newsgroup and would be a violation of netiquette. Anyone posting such a message would be flamed, embarrassed, ignored, or otherwise driven away. Your research responsibilities include searching for opposing views by visiting a variety of newsgroups and Web sites. A help here is to fall back on the familiar questions of journalism: who, what, when, where, and why.

- **Who** else might speak knowledgeably on this subject? Enter that person's name into a search engine. You might be surprised to find whose work is represented on the Web. (For fun, one of the authors entered the name of a rock-and-roll New York radio disk jockey into MetaCrawler and was amazed to find several pages devoted to the DJ, including sound clips of broadcasts dating back to the sixties, along with a history of his theme song.)

- **What** event might shed more information on your topic? Is there a group or organization that represents your topic? Do they hold an annual conference? Are synopses of presentations posted on the sponsoring organization's Web site?

- **When** do events happen? Annual meetings or seasonal occurrences can help you isolate newsgroup postings of interest.

- **Where** might you find this information? If you're searching for information on wines, for example, check to see if major wine-producing regions, such as the Napa Valley in California or the Rhine Valley in Germany, sponsor Web sites. These may point you to organizations or information that don't show up in other searches. Remember, Web search engines are fallible; they don't find every site you need.

- **Why** is the information you're searching for important? The answer to this question can lead you to related fields. New drugs, for example, are important not only to victims of diseases but to drug companies and the FDA as well.

part

1

Approach assertions you read from a skeptic's point of view. See if they stand up to critical evaluation or if you're merely emotionally attached to them. Imagine "What if . . . ?" or "What about . . . ?" scenarios that may disprove or at least call into question what you're reading. Try following each assertion you pull from the Internet with the phrase, "On the other hand. . . ." Because you can't leave the sentence hanging, you'll be forced to finish it, and this will help get you into the habit of critically examining information.

These are, of course, the same techniques critical thinkers have employed for centuries, only now you are equipped with more powerful search tools than past researchers may have ever imagined. In the time it took your antecedents to formulate their questions, you can search dozens of potential information sources. You belong to the first generation of college students to enjoy both quantity and quality in its research, along with a wider perspective on issues and the ability to form personal opinions after reasoning from a much wider knowledge base. Certainly, the potential exists for the Internet to grind out a generation of intellectual robots, "thinkers" who don't think but who regurgitate information from many sources. Technology always has its good and bad aspects. However, we also have the potential to become some of the most well-informed thinkers in the history of the world, thinkers who are not only articulate but confident that their opinions have been distilled from a range of views, processed by their own personalities, beliefs, and biases. This is one of the aspects of the Internet that makes this era such an exciting combination of humanism and technology.

part

1

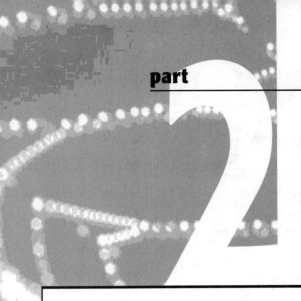

Health Related Activities on the Web

In this section you will find some activities that will help you use health related Internet Web sites in interesting and creative ways. Each of the activities will help you become more familiar with the Internet. They will also help you learn useful and unique ways to find excellent health information. These activities correspond with the health topic areas in the Address Book section of this text. You may find it helpful to refer back to these sections while doing the activities.

Activities

Health News

Something wonderful about the Internet is the speed with which information travels to and from all parts of the world. The research and developments that formerly took weeks and months to learn about are now available almost immediately. This activity will help you understand how this works.

First, go to the Health News page at the URL **http://www.siu.edu/ departments/bushea/news.html** Try to see how many news articles or news clips you can find that have come out in the past week or two on the topic of heart disease. How many of those news stories discuss

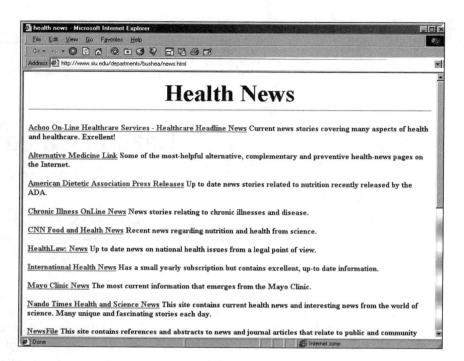

modes of treatment? How many describe ways to prevent heart disease? How many discuss risk factors for heart disease?

Do the same exercise for the following topics:

- Cancer
- HIV/AIDS
- Diabetes

Health Related Searches

This exercise will help you to become more proficient at using the search engines to your advantage. You may begin this exercise by going to the health search page **http://www.siu.edu/departments/bushea/search.html** Sexually transmitted diseases are a major health concern. Using the search engines on this page, find Web sites that give up-to-date information on the various types of sexually transmitted diseases that are common today. Look for current information on the following for each of the STDs:

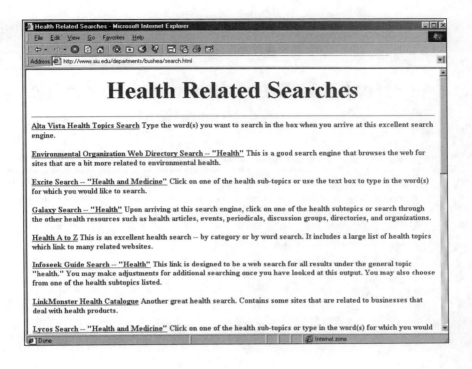

- Signs and symptoms
- Incubation periods of each
- Prevalence
- Treatment—which are curable, which aren't and how the curable are cured
- Prevention

For extra points, find pages with pictures of the various STDs, download them and include them in your graphics folder on your computer to be used in your next report on sexually transmitted diseases.

Health Related Journals, Magazines, and Periodicals

The next time one of your teachers gives you an assignment to do a health report, try to draw primarily from these online periodicals listed in the section of Journals, Magazines, and Periodicals: **http://www.siu. edu/departments/bushea/journal.html** Do not use them exclusively but

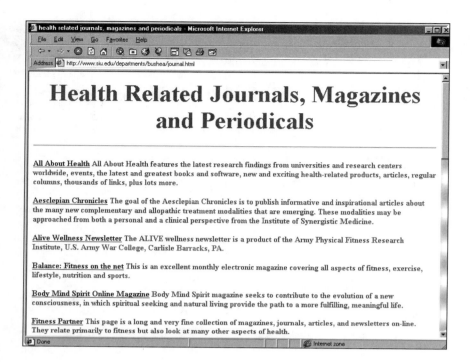

try to gather your information predominantly from these. See if the quality of the content of your paper is as good as the quality of those who use regular magazines, journals, and books to do theirs.

Health Research

Doing research on health topics can be unpleasant. The Internet has made the task of finding research easier. Although all research journals are not online, many journals' articles can be accessed from some of the research-based search engines. Medline is an example. To do a health research search, first go to **http://www.siu.edu/departments/bushea/ research.html** Next, click on **medline** to go to a medline search page. Once there, type a word or words in the text box that you want to research. Medline will bring up a list of related articles. You may choose one of these articles to see a complete abstract. If you have any questions, click the question mark in the upper right part of the Medline screen to improve your search.

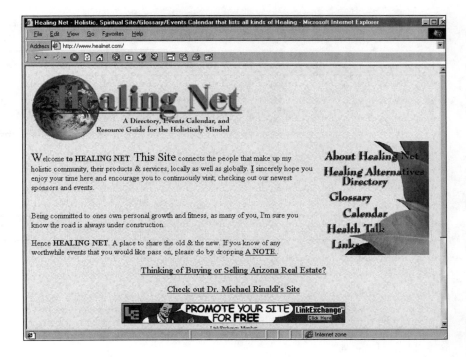

part

2

Alternative Medicine and Holistic Health

This exercise will help you gain a greater understanding of non-traditional or alternative forms of health and healing. In western medicine, we commonly treat headaches by taking an aspirin or some other type of pain reliever. However, there are other ways of treating the same problem without the use of drugs such as biofeedback, massage, acupressure or herbs. Go to the Healing Net Web Page at **http://www. healnet.com/** Using this page as a beginning point, find several alternative methods of treating the following maladies:

Muscle pain

_____

_____

Arthritis

_____

_____

Constipation

_____

_____

Stress

_____

_____

Cancer

_____

_____

Heart Disease

_____

_____

Others

_____

_____

Cancer

This exercise will help you become more acquainted with cancer information. Try to find answers to the following questions using this marvelous cancer information page called CanSearch located at **http://www.cansearch.org/canserch/canserch.htm**

Which type of cancer is the most prevalent in our society?

_____

_____

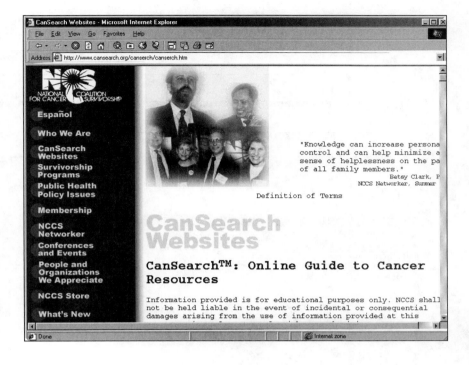

part
2

Which cancer has the greatest recovery rate?

_____

_____

Which type of cancer is usually the most painful?

_____

_____

Why is lung cancer such a dangerous form of cancer?

_____

_____

What are the best ways for women to decrease their risk of breast cancer?

_____

_____

What are the best ways for men to decrease their risk of prostate cancer?

_____

_____

What are the most common unconventional methods of cancer treatment?

_____

_____

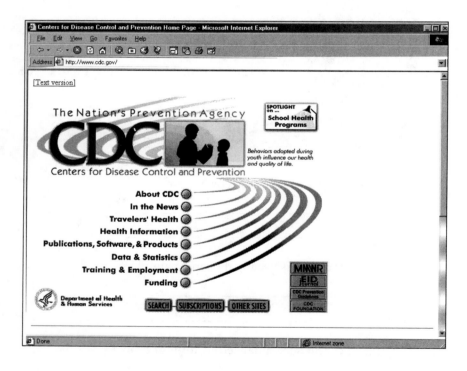

Community Health

This exercise will help you gather current information on community health issues that face our society. The Centers for Disease Control (CDC) has an excellent Web site for all things relating to the health of our communities and society. Using the CDC's Web site **http://www. cdc.gov/** find the answers to the following questions:

Which states in the country have the highest rates for the following:

    percentage of the population who exercise   _____

    percentage who smoke   _____

    percentage who are either overweight or obese   _____

    number of AIDS cases by state   _____

Comparing men and women, describe the cancer incidence and cancer deaths by sites in the body (e.g., breast, colon, lung)

_____

_____

part

2

How healthy is the water we drink and air we breathe in different parts of the country?

_____

_____

What are the leading causes of death in the U.S. for the following age groups:

    infants _____

    children _____

    adolescents _____

    young adults _____

    adults _____

    elderly _____

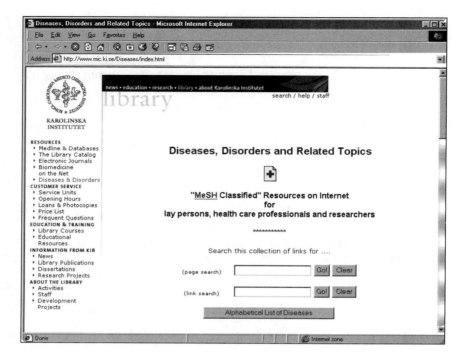

part

2

Diseases: Chronic and Acute

There are over 4,000 diseases known to exist in our society. Given the vast number and variety of diseases and illnesses, making sense of them can be quite a task. One Web site, The Karolinska Institute Library of Diseases and Disorders has put together a very impressive collection of most of the diseases of today. Go to this site by typing in the URL **http://www.mic.ki.se/Diseases/index.html** and use it to answer these questions (or any others that come to mind while you are searching through this Web site.

What are the common respiratory diseases in our society?

_____

_____

_____

What are the common signs and symptoms of respiratory diseases?

_____

_____

_____

What are the main causes for these types of diseases?

_____

_____

_____

What treatments are available for respiratory diseases?

_____

_____

_____

part
2

What are some common congenital diseases in our society?

_____

_____

_____

What are causes and treatments for these?

_____

_____

_____

This is an activity to learn more about how the immune system works. Using a metaphor, such as the sport of football, describe the immune system. Give the different parts of the immune system names that would apply in your metaphor. In the case of football, for example, the defensive line might be the T or B lymphocytes. What part of the immune system would be the linebackers? What about the tight end, the defensive backs and the cornerbacks? Would the coaches play a role? How would the offensive positions on a football team represent other parts of the immune system? Be creative.

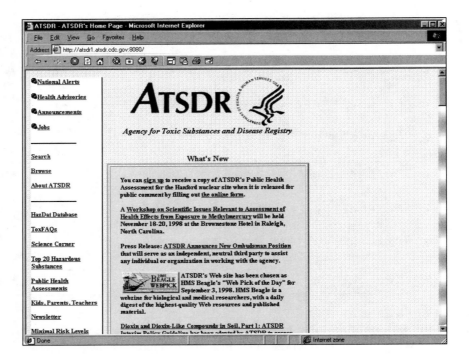

part

2

Environmental Health

Using the environmental health Web site, the Agency for Toxic Sub-
stances and Disease Registry, you will find the answers to these and
many other questions relating to our environment. Go to this Web site
by typing in the URL **http://atsdr1.atsdr.cdc.gov:8080/**

What is the ozone layer?

_____

_____

_____

What is the current state of the ozone?

_____

_____

_____

What are some common ways that we contaminate our water supply?

_____

_____

_____

What does the Safe Drinking Water Act of 1974 say?

_____

_____

_____

What are the most common sources of smog or air pollution in most cities?

_____

_____

_____

What are some common health effects of smog or air pollution?

_____

_____

_____

Who are the major polluters in your community?

_____

_____

_____

What kinds of chemicals are they releasing?

_____

_____

_____

Of these chemicals, which are the most dangerous?

_____

_____

_____

part

2

How many pounds of the most dangerous chemicals are they releasing?

_____

_____

Where is your state listed in the Toxic Release Inventory ranking?

_____

_____

How does your county compare with others in your state for the release of these chemicals?

_____

_____

_____

part

2

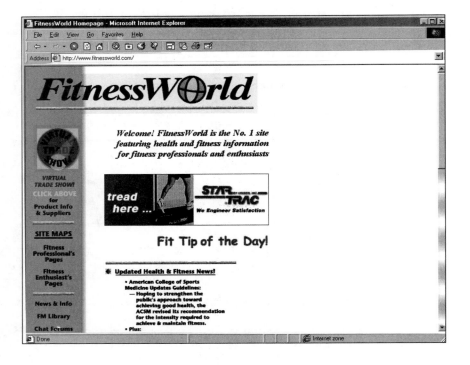

Exercise and Fitness

Few things we do can have more of a positive effect on our health than exercise. Attaining higher levels of activity and fitness is well known to be very beneficial. Go to FitnessWorld at the Web site **http://www. fitnessworld.com/** to find the answers to the following exercise questions:

What is your own aerobic exercise training zone based on your age?

_____

_____

_____

What are the recommended guidelines for aerobic activity for you?

_____

_____

_____

part

2

What is the best weight training program for you to enhance your exercise/activity program?

_____

_____

_____

When is the best time to stretch out and what are some good stretches for you based on the types of activity you participate in?

_____

_____

_____

General Health

The Web site, You First, at **http://www.youfirst.com/** contains a health risk appraisal. This health risk assessment includes all major factors relating to prevention and death: exercise, nutrition, smoking, alcohol use,

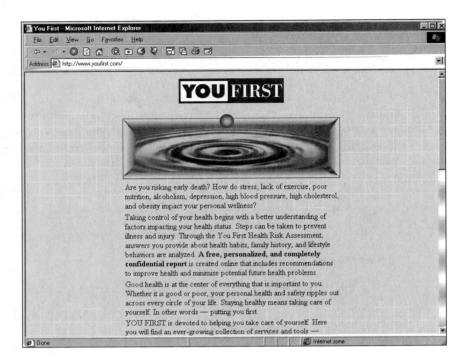

weight, cholesterol, blood pressure, back pain, vehicle safety, stress, depression, and cancer. Once you've answered all appropriate questions, click on the "results" button to receive your personalized health report. Your health assessment will be calculated and a customized Web page containing your results will be built. Review your health assessment, and take note of how you can make each day count toward building a healthier life. Based on the results of your health risk appraisal, how would you answer the following questions?

Are there current health conditions or habits that may lead to future health problems?

_____

_____

_____

Are there actions you can take to avoid health problems?

_____

_____

_____

In what ways can you improve and protect your health?

_____

_____

_____

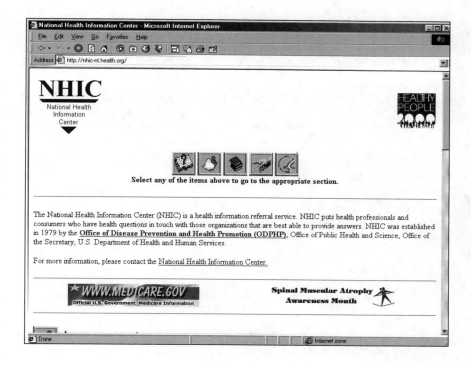

Government and Non-Government Health Resources and Databases

Here is an activity designed to help you find information on virtually any health related *organization* in this country and many others around the world. If you are unaware of where to begin your search, there are several Web sites that have started the process for you. The first one is **http://nhic-nt.health.org/** Once there, click on the words "Toll free numbers for health information." Immediately you will see an enormous list of health related organizations. Clicking on any of these will bring up an information page on that specific organization including how to contact them "toll free."

You will probably find what you are looking for by choosing the Yahoo! search for health associations. The address for this is **http://www.yahoo.com/Health/Organizations/**

With these two sites and a small investment of time, you can easily find information on just about any common, and some uncommon, health organizations that exist. You may also simply type in the words "health" and "organization" in the text box of any of your favorite search engines.

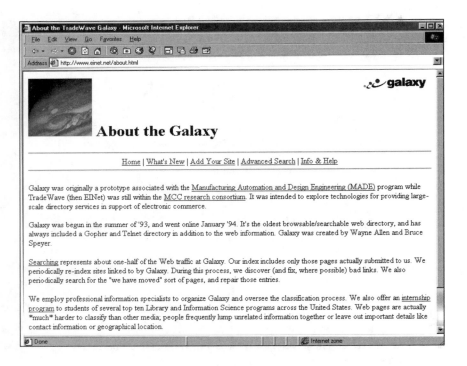

Health Education

Search through the Web site called Galaxy Search at **http://www.einet.net/about.html** Find three areas in community health that you are interested in. Then list several ways that health educators can play a key role to promote better health in these areas.

1. _____

    1. _____

    2. _____

    3. _____

2. _____

    1. _____

    2. _____

    3. _____

3. _____

    1. _____

    2. _____

    3. _____

part

2

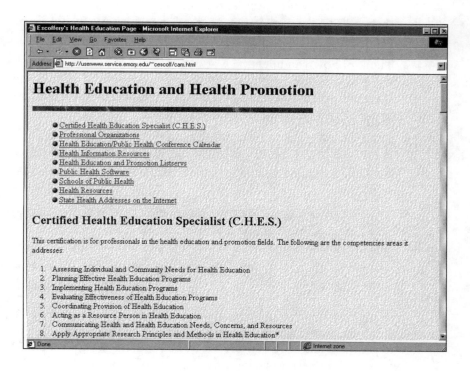

Health Psychology

A basic principle in health psychology is that of modeling. Modeling is one of the quickest ways of becoming very good at something. It involves finding someone else who has succeeded in doing that thing and doing the same things he or she did. This can be especially useful for beginning or intermediate health educators and health profession students. A nice activity designed to help you clarify where you want to go professionally follows a format something like this: (For this activity you will need a pen and a paper at first.)

1. Think of an area in health that interests you and write it down. (This may be quite broad such as fitness, or it may be more detailed such as a weight control specialist.)

2. Think of a setting that you would like to be working in once you are finished with your degree and write it down. (The majority of the health settings where health professionals work include the following: the worksite, the medical setting, the community, the school, or the university. There are many variations among these main settings.)

3. Think of how you might be working in that setting. What would you like your major roles to be? Write these down. (This might include something like managing a staff of aerobic instructors as part of a worksite health promotion program.)

4. Think of some ways you may be involved in assessing the needs of the setting. (How might you determine the types of health related activities and programs that will be appropriate for this particular setting?)

5. Think of some ways you may evaluate the effectiveness of your program. (For example, if it is a weight loss program, what amount of weight will the people need to lose and over how much time will they have to keep the pounds off in order for you to feel like your program is successful?)

Now, having generated these thoughts in your mind, your next step is to find the people who are doing the same things and learn what they did to get there and why they are successful at doing what they do. This is where the Internet can be a very valuable tool. One excellent starting place in this search might be the following URL **http://userwww.**

part

2

service.emory.edu/~cescoff/cam.html This page contains excellent information regarding the profession of health education. This includes professional certification, Health Education and Promotion Listservs or discussion groups, and State Health Addresses on the Internet. By subscribing to one of the listservs or accessing one of the professional organizations, you can quickly bring yourself into contact with many health professionals. You may also use any of your favorite search engines and type in the words "health" and "professional preparation." See what results come up and scroll through them. Once you find the person, there is usually a place where you can contact them using either email, snail mail or even a phone call. Finding the experts and the successful people in your field is that easy.

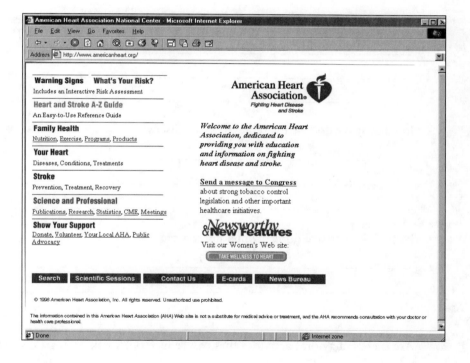

part

2

Heart Health

This exercise will help you become more acquainted with the number one killer in our society—heart disease. Answer the following questions using the Heart Health Web site from the American Heart Association. The URL for this Web site is **http://www.americanheart.org/**

What are the various types of heart disease?

_____

_____

_____

Can you find the average dollar costs of the various types of treatment currently available for heart disease?

_____

_____

_____

What is angina pectoris?

_____

_____

_____

part

2

In what ways does stress relate to heart disease?

_____

_____

_____

How does a stroke differ from a heart attack?

_____

_____

_____

Are there behavioral activities that can reduce one's risk of heart disease?

_____

_____

_____

The browser window shows:

Injury Control Resource Information Network

Check out ICRIN's new News Clipping Service

Please welcome ICRIN's new **Co-WebMaster:**
Gerald McGwin Jr., M.S, Ph.D.

NEW   Main Menu

Your Global Road Map to Internet Resources for Injury Control

Sponsored by the   *Center for Violence & Injury Control* **(CVIC)**   *Updated: 08/10/98*

part **2**

Injury Prevention and Safety

Do you know what to do if someone begins bleeding? What if someone begins to have a pain in their chest and down their left side? How do you respond to someone who has a tick stuck in their leg or has swallowed some poison? Look through the Injury Prevention page Injury Control Resource Information Network to find the answers to these and many other questions relating to first aid and injury prevention. The URL for this site is **http://www.injurycontrol.com/icrin/index.html**

Nutrition and Weight Control

For this exercise, first think of your favorite dinner at your favorite fast food restaurant. Write down each item on a piece of paper (For example: a Wendy's double hamburger with cheese, Biggie fries, large Frosty, and a cookie). Using the Fast Food Finder Web site at **http://www. olen.com/food/** find the following information:

What is the total number of calories for the meal? _____

What is the total number of fat calories for the meal? _____

What is the total number of saturated fat calories? _____

What is the percentage of fat calories for the meal? _____

What is the percentage of saturated fat calories? _____

What is the total number of simple sugar (simple carbohydrate) calories? _____

How does your meal stack up with current recommendations for good nutrition?

_____

_____

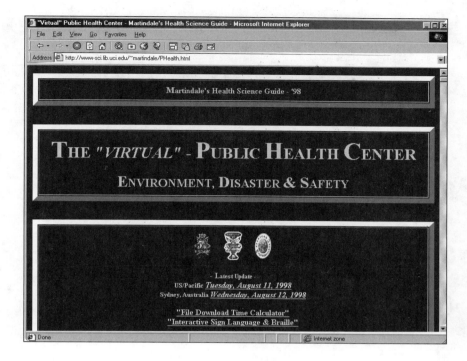

Public Health

Here is a little activity that will thoroughly amaze you. I promise. First type in the following Web site in your browser's URL window **http://www-sci.lib.uci.edu/~martindale/PHealth.html** This Web site is called *The Virtual Public Health Center.* You will find that you can easily spend a few minutes or a few hours at this one location. Just look through all the variety of activities and information relating not only to public health, but to a host of other subjects that are health related. This is one of the finest Web sites out there. Stop in for a visit. You will not be disappointed!

Self-Help and Self-Care

You have a relative who suffers from chemical hypersensitivity or environmental illness. Using Health World OnLine at

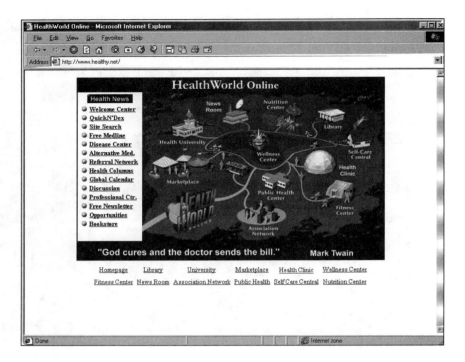

http://www.healthy.net/, find at least three different support groups or agencies where she can go for help.

1. _____

2. _____

3. _____

Stress Management

Stress affects us all, but not in the same ways. For this reason, we must have many ways to manage and reduce our stress before it adversely affects us. Experts say that sixty to ninety percent of hospital admissions have a stress component. For this activity, go to the stress management Web site titled "Relax.Calm." The URL for this wonderful Web site is **http://www.concord.wvnet.edu/~olpin/relax.html**

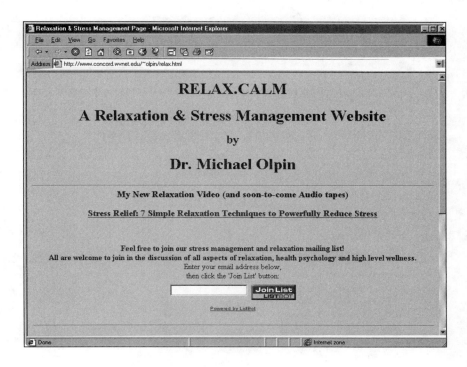

Using the information from this page and the links to other excellent stress management places, list 5 ways that you could effectively reduce the amount of stress in your life.

1. _____

2. _____

3. _____

4. _____

5. _____

Tobacco, Alcohol, and Drug Use

Go to the National Clearinghouse Prevline at **http://www.health.org/aboutn** Click on home page at the bottom of the introductory page. Now click on Alcohol and Drug Facts. Using this information find out how many drinks it takes for you to reach certain blood alcohol levels.

part

2

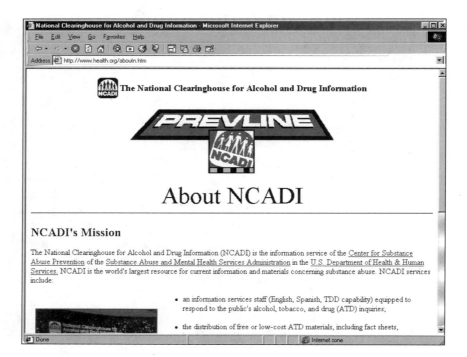

part
2

How much alcohol constitutes one drink? What are the effects on your driving and decision making abilities after two drinks?

You have a friend who may have a problem with alcohol or drugs. Proceed to **http://www.health.org/pubs/strafact/straight.htm#signs2** Go over the checklist provided, making note of the areas that pertain to your friend. Then find several referrals to help your friend with this problem.

1. _____

2. _____

3. _____

Violence Resources and Information

Using the Web site Domestic Violence: The Facts at **http://www.igc.apc.org/fund/the_facts/** answer the following quiz questions.

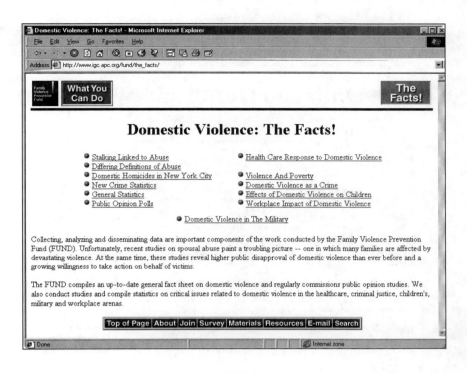

part

2

1. True or False   In a comparison of delinquent and nondelinquent youth it was found that a history of violence or abuse is the most significant difference between the two groups.

2. What percentage of murdered women are killed by their intimate male partners?

   35%   42%   52%

3. Of the 143 accredited U.S. and Canadian medical schools, what percentage of schools do not require their medical students to receive instruction about domestic violence?

   53%   63%   73%

4. Since the television coverage of the O. J. Simpson case, have Americans become more or less active in doing something about domestic violence? Why?

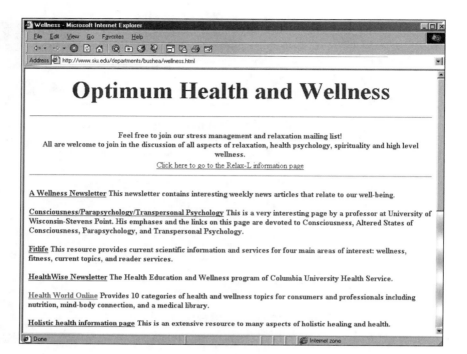

Wellness and Optimum Health

Based on the information found in the Wellness and Optimum Health resource sites at **http://www.siu.edu/departments/bushea/wellness.html**, create your own health newsletter.

Design the letter around your specific interests in health. You may want to include local community health information, pictures, and health articles. After creating the newsletter, print several copies and distribute them to your friends, family, or coworkers. You may even want to distribute them to community members in your area.

Women's Health

You have a friend who has just discovered she is pregnant. She is interested in learning about her childbirth options. Using the Internet page Med Web Gynecology and women's health at **http://www.gen.**

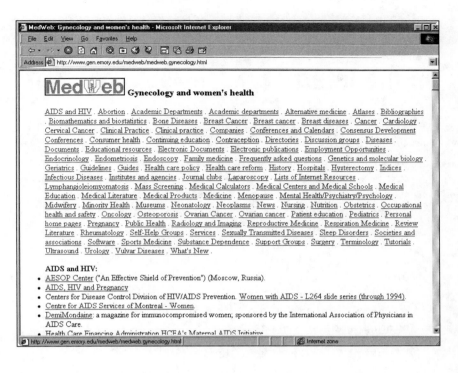

emory.edu/medweb/medweb.gynecology.html, help her identify her options.

Also help her answer the following:

1. What are the differences between midwives and obstetricians?

2. What should she know about delivering in a hospital, a birthing center, or at home?

3. What other options does she have?

4. Should she exercise during pregnancy?

5. What are common complications resulting from pregnancy?

6. What routine tests will she be given and what do the results mean?

7. What are five more sources, support groups, or agencies she can contact for further information?

part

2

Health Related Web Sites on the Internet

This section is filled with Web sites related to all aspects of health. Each site is listed first with the URL (Universal Resource Locator) which is the Internet address. These addresses must be typed in your browser's URL text box exactly as they are shown. If any part of the URL is missing, you will not arrive where you want to go. The second part of the listings below is the title for each Web site. This is followed by a short description of what is to be found at the particular Web site.

One thing is sure about the Internet—it is in a constant state of change. All of the Web sites listed in this book were functioning at the time of publication. The Web sites that were selected for this book are ones that have been quite stable over the past few years.

Every listing in this book can also be accessed from the following health promotion Web page:

`http://www.siu.edu/departments/bushea/`

You can save yourself some time by creating a "bookmark" to this page using your web browser.

The Web sites that follow are categorized first by the following topics: Health News, Health Related Internet Searches, Health Related Journals, Magazines, and Periodicals, and Health Research and Evaluation. These are followed by the following health content areas: alternative medicine and holistic health; cancer; community health; diseases; environmental health; exercise and fitness; general health; health and disease care; health education; health promotion; health psychology; heart health; food and nutrition; public health; safety and injury prevention; self-help and self-care; stress management; tobacco, alcohol and drug use; violence; weight control; wellness and optimum health; and women's health.

part

2

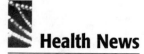

Health News

Achoo On-Line

`http://www.achoo.com/features/headlinenews/index.htm`

Healthcare Services—Healthcare Headline News. News stories covering many aspects of health and healthcare. Excellent!

Alternative Medicine Link

http://www.altmedicine.com/

Some of the most helpful alternative, complementary, and preventive health-news pages on the Internet.

American Dietetic Association Press Releases

http://www.eatright.org/pressindex.html

Up-to-date news stories related to nutrition recently released by the ADA.

Chronic Illness OnLine News

http://www.chronicillnet.org/online/

News stories relating to chronic illnesses and disease.

CNN Food and Health News

http://www.cnn.com/HEALTH/index.html

Recent news regarding nutrition and health from science.

HealthLaw: News

http://www.ljextra.com/practice/health/index.html

Up-to-date news on national health issues from a legal point of view.

Mayo Clinic News

http://www.mayohealth.org/ivi/mayo/common/htm/
newsstnd.htm

The most current information that emerges from the Mayo Clinic.

Nando Times Health and Science News

http://www.nando.net/nt/health/index_t.html

This site contains current health news and interesting news from the world of science. Many unique and fascinating stories each day.

part
2

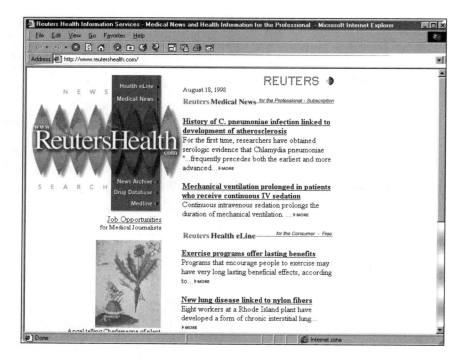

NewsPage Health and Healthcare News Stories

http://www.newspage.com/NEWSPAGE/cgi-bin/walk.cgi/
NEWSPAGE/info/d15/

A topically guided page filled with health articles that are more medical
and disease-care oriented.

Reuters Health Information Services

http://www.reutershealth.com/

Daily news stories on health and disease. This is an excellent "first stop"
for daily health news divided into news topics for the health professional
and health consumer.

The News-Times Health News

http://www.newstimes.com/news/today/health.htm

This is another daily news stories page that lists headline health
stories.

USA Today Health

`http://www.usatoday.com/life/health/lhd1.htm`

Health news stories from USA today.

Wellness Newsletter

`http://www.wellmedia.com/news.html`

Weekly stories and articles mostly on items that are wellness related.

Yahoo! Health News Daily

`http://www.yahoo.com/headlines/health/`

Yahoo!'s news section on daily health stories. Another excellent "first stop" for daily health news.

Your Health Daily

`http://nytsyn.com/med/`

Daily health related news stories from the New York Times.

Health Related Searches

Alta Vista Health Topics Search

`http://www.altavista.digital.com/`

An excellent search engine. Just type the word(s) you want to search in the box.

Environmental Organization Web Directory Search—Health

`http://www.webdirectory.com/Health/`

This is a good search engine that browses the web for sites that are related to environmental health.

Excite Search—Health and Medicine

`http://my.excite.com/lifestyle/health_and_fitness/`

Click on one of the health sub-topics or use the text box to type in the word(s) for which you would like to search.

part

2

Galaxy Search—Health

`http://www.einet.net/galaxy/Community/Health.html`

Upon arriving at this search engine, click on one of the health subtopics or search through the other health resources such as health articles, events, periodicals, discussion groups, directories, and organizations.

Health A to Z

`http://www.HealthAtoZ.com/`

This is an excellent health search—by category or by word search. It includes a large list of health topics which link to many related Web sites.

Infoseek Guide Search—Health

`http://guide-p.infoseek.com/Health?tid=1207`

This link is designed to be a web search for all results under the general topic of health. You may make adjustments for additional searching once you have looked at this output. You may also choose from one of the health subtopics listed.

LinkMonster Health Catalogue

`http://www.linkmonster.com/health.html`

Another great health search. Contains some sites that are related to businesses that deal with health products.

Lycos Search—Health and Medicine

`http://a2z.lycos.com/Health_and_Medicine/`

Click on one of the health sub-topics or type in the word(s) for which you would like to search.

Magellan Search—Health and Medicine

`http://www.mckinley.com/magellan/Reviews/`
`Health_and_Medicine/index.magellan.html`

Click on one of the health sub-topics or type in the word(s) for which you would like to search.

part

2

Medicle Matrix

http://www.medmatrix.org/index.asp

This search engine is a guide to Internet Clinical Medicine Resources. It is a HUGE Resource for medicine and disease care.

Virtual Hospital

http://vh.radiology.uiowa.edu/Misc/Search.html

With this search engine, simply type the keyword(s) in the box. This engine is designed to be more medically oriented.

WebCrawler Health Topics Search

http://webcrawler.com/Health/

Choose from one of the displayed topics or click search and type in the health topic that you seek.

Yahoo! Search—Health

http://www.yahoo.com/Health/

This site allows you to use the popular Yahoo! search engine to seek health information. Choose one of the health categories listed or type a subject in the box and then click the search button next to the text box.

part
2

Health Related Journals, Magazines, and Periodicals

All About Health

http://www.allabouthealth.com/

All About Health features the latest research findings from universities and research centers worldwide, events, the latest and greatest books and software, new and exciting health related products, articles, regular columns, thousands of links, plus lots more.

Aesclepian Chronicles

http://www.forthrt.com/~chronicl/homepage.html

The goal of the Aesclepian Chronicles is to publish informative and inspirational articles about the many new complementary and allopathic treatment modalities that are emerging. These modalities may be approached from both a personal and a clinical perspective from the Institute of Synergistic Medicine.

Alive Wellness Newsletter

http://carlisle-www.army.mil/apfri/alive.htm

The ALIVE wellness newsletter is a product of the Army Physical Fitness Research Institute, U.S. Army War College, Carlisle Barracks, PA.

Balance: Fitness on the Net

part 2

http://ww2.hyperlink.com/balance/

This is an excellent monthly electronic magazine covering all aspects of fitness, exercise, lifestyle, nutrition, and sports.

Body Mind Spirit Online Magazine

http://www.hinman.oro.net/~bmsweb/bmsmag.htm

Body Mind Spirit magazine seeks to contribute to the evolution of a new consciousness in which spiritual seeking and natural living provide the path to a more fulfilling, meaningful life.

Fitness Partner

http://primusweb.com/fitnesspartner/

This page is a long and very fine collection of magazines, journals, articles, and newsletters online. They relate primarily to fitness but also look at many other aspects of health.

Lifelines Newsletter

http://www.lifelines.com/lifenews.html

A publication that encourages better health and a better life.

Mayo Clinic Newsletter On-Line

http://healthnet.ivi.com/ivi/mayo/common/htm/
library.htm

Monthly articles and news items. Very timely articles from the Mayo clinic.

Medscape

http://www.medscape.com/

For health professionals and interested consumers, this newsletter features thousands of full-text, peer-reviewed articles, medical news, Medline, and interactive quizzes. Updated daily, and Free!

Men's Fitness On-Line

http://mensfitness.com/

Online rendition of the magazine bearing the same name.

New Frontier: Magazine of Transformation

http://www.newfrontier.com/

Monthly editions of an online newsletter dedicated to promoting high levels of health and wellness.

part

2

New Age Journal On-Line

http://www.newage.com/

New Age Journal is committed to uncovering traditional wisdom and integrating it with modern technology. New Age Journal provides more than merely simple information. It is a magazine of insight and perspective, covering people and issues often ignored by the mainstream, and uncovering trends not yet discovered by the more popular press.

New England Journal of Medicine On-line

http://www.nejm.org/

This is a weekly journal reporting the results of important medical research worldwide.

Nutrition Action Healthletter

http://www.cspinet.org/nah/

A health letter published by the Center for Science in the Public Interest.

One excellent list of Health Journals and Periodicals

http://pie.org/E21221T3783

Here is another list of online health and medical journals.

The Physician and Sports Medicine Online

http://www.physsportsmed.com/

This Web site features abstracts from the current issue of the magazine, actual articles from previous issues, a search feature to find selected topics from back issues, and a Personal Health section with patient-oriented articles on exercise, nuitrition and injury prevention.

Self-Help and Psychology Magazine

http://www.well.com/user/selfhelp/index.html

A self-help resource that includes articles; self-help book reviews; movie reviews and software reviews for parents; questions and answers written by professionals; an interactive corner; cartoons; links, lists, and newsgroups spanning mental-health sites across the globe; a full-service bookstore; professional information and services, and much more. Go in and help yourself!

The Share Guide Holistic Health Journal and Directory

http://www.shareguide.com/mag/

This is a magazine focusing on holistic health, personal growth and environmental awareness.

Yoga Journal

http://www.yogajournal.com/

This is a is a journal dedicated to communicating to as broad an audience as possible, the qualities of being that yoga exemplifies: peace, integrity, clarity, and compassion.

Health Research and Evaluation

Carl Uncover

http://www.carl.org/Access.html

Search the largest set of licensed databases in the industry, from local and national newspapers to outstanding sources in business, sciences, technology, medicine, social sciences, the arts, consumer information, patents, education and reference sources, along with the online public access catalog and any Z39.50 library catalog on the web.

Combined Health Information Database

http://chid.nih.gov/

CHID is a database produced by health-related agencies of the Federal Government. This database provides titles, abstracts, and availability information for health information and health education resources. The value of this database is that it lists a wealth of health promotion and education materials and program descriptions that are not indexed elsewhere. New records are added quarterly and current listings are checked regularly to help ensure that all entries are up to date and still available from their original sources. Some older records are retained for archival purposes.

part

2

Eric Clearinghouse on Assessment and Evaluation

http://ericae.net/

Eric looks for journal articles that are a bit more related but not limited to education.

Healthfinder On-line Publications

http://www.healthfinder.gov/moretools/

Many of the best federal consumer health information publications available online are included in the healthfinder database. Search for online publications, publications catalogs, and Web sites featuring electronic documents.

Health Services Research/Public Health Journals

http://weber.u.washington.edu/~hserv/authinst/
jolist.html

This site contains an exhausive list of research journals that are considered to be useful to health services research/public health practitioners. It contains enhanced links including tables of content and subscription information.

Medline

http://www.healthgate.com/HealthGate/MEDLINE/
search.shtml

Search through Medline for peer-reviewed journal articles on most aspects of health and disease.

NewsFile

http://www.homepage.holowww.com/

This site contains references and abstracts to news and journal articles that relate to public and community health. An excellent resource for research.

NYU Health Education Professional Resources

http://www.nyu.edu/education/hepr/resources/online/
index.html

This page contains another excellent list of links to health related research resources online.

Ovid Technologies

http://www.ovid.com/

Platform-independent access to bibliographic and live full text databases for academic, biomedical and scientific research.

PsychJournal Search

http://www.cmhc.com/journals/

This page contains a searchable index of 1,000+ psychology and social science journals online.

Community Health Research Methods Practitioner's Home Page

http://web.indstate.edu/hlthsfty/hlth341/home.htm

Steve Gabeny's excellent online research and evaluation course.

The Web as a Research Tool: Evaluation Techniques

http://www.science.widener.edu/~withers/evalout.htm

Provides opportunities to critique the WWW as a source of information. Fosters critical thinking skills with online instruction on how to evaluate.

part

2

Alternative Medicine and Holistic Health

Acupuncture.com

http://www.Acupuncture.com/

Traditional oriental therapies along with related resources for consumers, practitioners, and students. Includes other related information and links as well.

Alternative Medicine Homepage

http://www.pitt.edu/~cbw/altm.html

A jumpstation for sources of information on unconventional, unorthodox, unproven, or alternative, complementary, innovative, and integrative therapies.

Alternative Medicine Links

http://www.altmedicine.com/

Some of the most-helpful alternative, complementary and preventive health-news pages on the Internet.

Alternative Medicine Weekly

http://www.rhemamed.com/altmed.htm

Studies conducted using alternative medicine are listed weekly from this excellent Web site. Drop in regularly.

The Amazing Maze of Natural Medicine

http://www.medicalmaze.com/index.html

This site contains very interesting articles and information on natural medicine.

The American Association of Naturopathic Physicians

http://healer.infinite.org/

This is an excellent resource on all things having to do with healing and martial arts.

American Massage Therapy Association

http://www.amtamassage.org/

The mission of the American Massage Therapy Association is to develop and advance the art, science and practice of massage therapy in a caring, professional and ethical manner in order to promote the health and welfare of humanity. Visit the site of this most popular form of complementary health care.

Buffalo Springboard

http://www.quake.net/~xdcrlab/hp.html

Links to sources of information, advice and articles for alternative health.

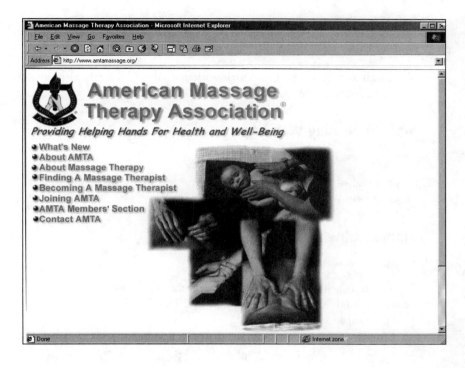

Dream Up, Dream Links

http://www.dreamup.com/

This site contains nearly everything you could want to know about the magical world of dreaming.

Herbal Information Center

http://www.kcweb.com/herb/herbmain.htm

Here, you will find descriptions of the most common herbs, and how they can be used to treat today's health problems.

HerbNET

http://www.herbnet.com/

This site claims to be the most comprehensive site on the Web for those seeking information on herbs, herb products and remedies, herb publications . . . in fact everything herbal can be found here!

Herb Research (Foundation) News

http://www.herbs.org/index.html

Research and education on worldwide use of herbs for health, environmental conservation, and international development.

Holistic Healing Web Page

http://www.holisticmed.com/

Extensive holistic health related information including articles, web links, group links and mailing information lists.

Homeopathy Home Page

http://www.homeopathyhome.com/

This page is a jumping off point and aims to provide links to every resource available related to homeopathy. There are FAQs, a reference library, discussion groups, etc.

part
2

Hot Links to the Best WWW Holistic Health Resources

http://www.samart.co.th/hps/wwwresor.htm

The title says it all.

HPS Online

http://login.samart.co.th/~hps/

This is another site that contains an extraordinary amount of very interesting holistic health information. They touch nearly every holistic base.

Interlude Links

http://www.nursery.com/~interlud/links.htm

Websites that are good for you!

The International Advocates for Health Freedom

http://www.iahf.com/

The creators of this page describe themselves as a catalytic entity designed to foster networking between health freedom activists worldwide in order to foster opposition to the elements of coercion: the UN's International Council of Drug Regulating Authorities, and all regulating bodies falling under its auspices including the FDA, TGA, HPB, MCA, MCC, etc.

The International Society for the Enhancement of Eyesight

`http://ezinfo.ucs.indiana.edu/~aeulenbe/i_see`

A Web site and contents of a mailing list dedicated to promoting better natural eyesight for everyone!

Medweb: Alternative Medicine

`http://www.gen.emory.edu/MEDWEB/keyword/`
`alternative_medicine.html`

Extensive resourse for links to information and sites for alternative medicine.

Natural Medicine, Complementary Health Care and Alternative Therapies

`http://www.teleport.com/~amrta/`

Links and resources for education in organizations, news, and programs for alternative medicine.

Office of Alternative Medicine at the National Institutes of Health

`http://altmed.od.nih.gov/`

Office of Alternative Medicine (OAM) identifies and evaluates unconventional health care practices. The OAM supports and conducts research and research training on these practices and disseminates information.

Oxygen and Ozone Therapies

`http://www.oxytherapy.com/`

Information on oxygen therapies including, the use of hydrogen peroxide, ozone therapy, hyperbaric oxygen, stabilized oxygen, and ionization.

part

2

Spirit WWW

http://www.spiritweb.org/

Spirituality Resources on the WWW including links to many forms of spirituality.

The Weaver Spirituality Page

http://ww2.hyperlink.com/weaver/

A page dedicated to spirituality, holistic health, religious and psychotherapeutic health. Written in article form by many different authors with new issues every month.

Wellness Links

http://wellmedia.com/links.html

Links to many Web sites relating to holistic thinking, spirituality, and personal development.

part

2

Cancer

American Cancer Society

http://www.cancer.org/

Official home page for the ACS concerning the symptoms, treatment, and prevention of cancer.

Breast Cancer Information Clearinghouse

http://nysernet.org/bcic/

A Web site designed to provide information for breast cancer patients and their families.

Cancer Care Inc.

http://www.cancercareinc.org/

This cancer related Web site lists Internet- and telephone-based support services, as well as information on counseling, local physicians referrals, and even financial assistance. Online forums allow patients to converse with experts.

Cancer News on the Net

http://www.cancernews.com/

This site is dedicated to bringing patients and their families the latest information on cancer diagnosis and treatment.

CanSearch

http://www.cansearch.org/canserch/canserch.htm

The purpose of this guide is to assist those not experienced in finding sources on the Net to go to cancer resources quickly and find answers to their questions or at least become more informed patients and caretakers.

InterNet Resources for Cancer

http://www.ncl.ac.uk/~nchwww/guides/clinks1.htm

This guide contains over 30 pages of links to cancer related information. Many sites contain information for both the public and health professionals.

JOMOL Cancer Research Information

http://africa.com/~martin/jomol/

Information on an alternative therapy for cancer.

National Cancer Institute

http://www.nci.nih.gov/

Complete information source of the National Cancer Institute. The National Cancer Institute (NCI) is a component of the National Institutes of Health (NIH), one of eight agencies that compose the Public Health Service (PHS) in the Department of Health and Human Services (DHHS). The NCI, established under the National Cancer Act of 1937, is the Federal Government's principal agency for cancer research and training.

part
2

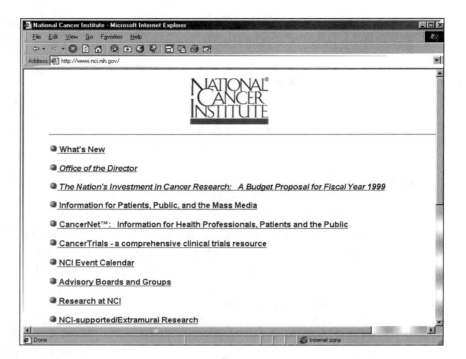

National Cancer Institutes' Comprehensive Cancer Database

http://cancernet.nci.nih.gov/pdq.htm

NCI's comprehensive cancer database, contains peer-reviewed statements on treatment, supportive care, prevention, and screening, as well as anti-cancer drugs; a registry of over 1,600 open and 8,000 closed clinical trials from around the world; and directories of physicians and organizations that provide cancer care, including more than 4,000 FDA-approved mammography screening facilities.

National Comprehensive Cancer Network

http://www.cancer.med.umich.edu/NCCN/NCCN.html

The NCCN was formed to create cancer-management strategies for large employers and third-party payers. Its mission is to integrate the experience of member cancer centers to ensure delivery of high-quality, cost-effective services to cancer patients across the country.

Skin Cancer Information Page

http://www.maui.net/~southsky/introto.html

A very through information page on skin cancer. Designed to be a gathering place for all available information about skin cancer and related subjects.

Steve Dunn's Cancer Information Page

http://cancerguide.org/

A very informative guide dedicated to helping you find the answers to your questions about cancer, and especially to helping you find the questions you need to ask.

University of Pennsylvania Cancer Resource

http://www.oncolink.upenn.edu/

An extensive Web site touted as the first multimedia oncology information resource placed on the Internet.

Yahoo!'s Cancer Links

http://www.yahoo.com/Health/Diseases_and_Conditions/Cancer/

A thorough search of the Internet's Web sites devoted to information on the various types of cancer.

part

2

Community Health Education

American Heart Association National Center

http://www.amhrt.org/

The American Heart Association is one of the world's premier health organizations, and is committed to reducing disability and death from cardiovascular diseases and stroke. This site provides a wealth of information with listings under almost 300 subjects.

Center for Disease Control and Prevention

http://www.cdc.gov/cdc.html

The CDC's mission is to promote health and quality of life by preventing and controlling disease, injury, and disability. This site contains links to other agencies, and a lot of information on various health related topics such as, the CDC, health information, travelers' health, publications and products, data and statistics, training and employment, and funding.

Community Health Concepts Home Page

http://web.indstate.edu/hlthsfty/ch/ch.htm

This page includes community health courses with outlines, excellent information, and a huge list of community health related links. This is a great resource.

Escoffery's Health Education Page

http://userwww.service.emory.edu/~cescoff/cam.html

A jumpsite to resources on Certified Health Education Specialist (C.H.E.S.), professional organizations, health education/public health conference calendar, health information resources, health education and promotion listservs, public health software, schools of public health, health resources, and state health addresses on the Internet.

National Health Information Center

http://nhic-nt.health.org/

NHIC is a health information referral service which puts health professionals and consumers who have health questions in touch with those organizations that are best able to provide answers. This is a great resource for health publications, announcements, and access to 1,100 health organizations and government offices.

National Institutes of Health

http://www.nih.gov/

Great information about the NIH, health information, news and events, grants and contracts, scientific research, and more.

Pan American Health Organization

http://www.paho.org/

PAHO's mission is to cooperate technically with the Member Countries and to stimulate cooperation among them in order that, while maintaining a healthy environment and charting a course to sustainable human development, the peoples of the Americas may achieve health for all and by all.

World Health Association

http://www.who.ch/

The objective of WHO is the attainment by all peoples of the highest possible level of health. Health, as defined in the WHO Constitution, is a state of complete physical, mental and social well-being and not merely the absence of disease or infirmity.

Diseases: Chronic and Acute

part
2

A2Z Search—Illness and Disorders

http://a2z.lycos.com/Health_and_Medicine/
Illnesses_and_Disorders/

A web search for information by disease categories using the engine called A2Z.

American Diabetes Association

http://www.diabetes.org/

This is the home page of the American Diabetes Association. Their mission is to prevent and cure diabetes and to improve the lives of all people affected by diabetes.

American Lung Association

http://www.lungusa.org/

This is the ALA online resource for information on asthma and other lung diseases, tobacco control, and environmental health.

CDC Diseases Page

http://www.cdc.gov/diseases/diseases.html

Information on many diseases in the United States including data on incidence and prevalence of diseases.

Chronic Illness-Net

http://www.chronicillnet.org/

This Web site describes itself as the first multimedia information source on the Internet dedicated to chronic illnesses including AIDS, cancer, Persian Gulf War Syndrome, autoimmune diseases, Chronic Fatigue Syndrome, heart disease, and neurological diseases.

Diseases, Disorders, and Related Topics

http://www.mic.ki.se/Diseases/index.html

part

2

Diseases, Disorders, and Related Topics catalogs resources on the Internet for laypersons, health care professionals, and scientists. A gigantic resource—excellent place to begin searching for disease information.

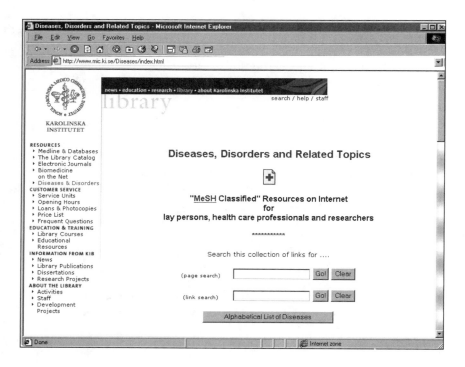

Med Help General Library

http://medhlp.netusa.net/

This page links to thousands (seemingly) of articles covering a wide variety of diseases, conditions, and health concerns.

Morbidity and Mortality Weekly Report

http://www.cdc.gov/epo/mmwr/mmwr.html

The Morbidity and Mortality Weekly Report (MMWR) Series is prepared by the Centers for Disease Control and Prevention (CDC) and is based on weekly reports to CDC by state health departments.

Mother Nature's General Store: Health Library

http://www.mothernature.com/hotlist.htm

A general health information library that includes information on AIDS and cancer.

part

2

National Center for Chronic Disease Prevention and Health Promotion

http://ftp.cdc.gov/nccdphp/nccdhome.htm

A page devoted to consolidating National Centers for Disease Control and Prevention (CDC) efforts in chronic disease prevention and health promotion.

On-Line Allergy Center

http://www.sig.net/~allergy/welcome.html

Browse through these pages for helpful information on the relief of a variety of symptoms including nasal congestion, eye redness/soreness, sneezing, wheezing, coughing, joint pain, intestinal pain, skin rashes/irritation, itching, yeast infections, mood swings, hyperactivity, attention deficit disorder, and fatigue.

Point Search's Top 5%

http://point.lycos.com/topics/Conditions_Overall.html

Point Communication lists and describes the top Web sites around the world that are disease related.

STD Home Page

http://med-www.bu.edu/people/sycamore/std/std.htm

This page is an excellent overview of the major STDs of our society. It includes some nice graphics and some excellent resources related to STDs.

Virology WWW server

http://www.bocklabs.wisc.edu/Welcome.html

This Web site is a huge resource collecting all possible information related to viruses including maps of viruses, digitized images of viruses, conferences, news and journals, links, emerging infectious diseases, and more.

Yahoo!: Diseases and Conditions

http://www.yahoo.com/Health/Diseases_and_Conditions/

Yahoo! search for Web sites on the Internet that are disease related.

part

2

Environmental Health

Agency for Toxic Substances and Disease Registry

http://atsdr1.atsdr.cdc.gov:8080/cx.html

A simple guide to search the World Wide Web for environmental health information. The primary focus is to find and share global information resources with the public on the linkage between human exposure to hazardous chemicals and adverse human health effects.

National Center for Environmental Health (NCEH)

http://www.cdc.gov/nceh/ncehhome.htm

The mission of the NCEH is to provide national leadership, through science and service, to promote health and quality of life by preventing and controlling disease, birth defects, disability, and death resulting from interactions between people and their environment.

National Institute of Environmental Health Sciences

http://www.niehs.nih.gov/

The mission of the National Institute of Environmental Health Sciences (NIEHS) is to reduce the burden of human illness and dysfunction from environmental causes by understanding each of these elements and how they interrelate.

Project NatureConnect

http://www.pacificrim.net/~nature/

This page is especially for nature enthusiasts. The designers of this page created this site to help others promote a profoundly heightened sense of self worth and environmental responsibility.

Yahoo! Search on Environmental Health

http://www.yahoo.com/Health/Environmental_Health/

Multiple sites, links, and home pages as well as information on environmental health.

part

2

Exercise and Fitness

American Academy of Family Physicians Foundation

http://research.med.umkc.edu/aafp/Q19.html

A database listing of favorably reviewed materials on exercise, fitness, and stress management.

American Alliance for Health, Physical Education, Recreation, and Dance

http://www.aahperd.org/

AAHPERD's home page includes links to American Association for Active Lifestyles and Fitness, American Association for Health Education, American Association for Leisure and Recreation, National Association for Girls and Women in Sport, National Association for Sport and Physical Education, and the National Dance Association.

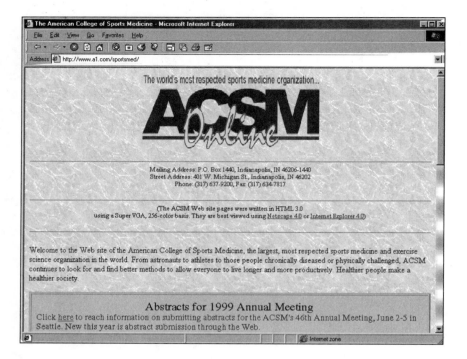

part

2

American College of Sports Medicine

http://www.a1.com/sportsmed/

This is the home page of the largest, most respected sports medicine and exercise science organization in the world.

American Council on Exercise

http://www.acefitness.org/

This not-for-profit organization sets certification standards for exercise professionals and runs a consumer fitness hotline offering referrals to ACE certified personal trainers. Their Web site features information about their programs, referrals to fitness resources and news about exercise and fitness.

Bicycling Information

http://www.cascade.org/links.html

This site is loaded with bicycling Web sites all over the world. Nearly anything you might want to know regarding bicycling can be accessed from this page.

Dr. Pribut's Running Injuries Page

http://www.clark.net/pub/pribut/spsport.html

This site contains information about running and about preventing and treating many types of running injuries.

FitnessLab

http://members.aol.com/ironmaan/fitnesslab.html

This great fitness site contains nutrition and fitness software, articles, and associated links.

Fitness Products Council

http://www.sportlink.com/fitness/

Contains a Speakers Bureau, market research reports, a newsletter, and the Surgeon General's recent report on health, fitness, and exercise.

Exercise, Fitness and Pregnancy

http://www.noah.cuny.edu/pregnancy/march_of_dimes/pre
_preg.plan/fit42is.html

A lot of information on excersise and pregnancy, including benefits, risks, and guidelines.

Exercise, Fitness, and Big Folks

http://www.comlab.ox.ac.uk/oucl/users/sharon.curtis/
BigFolks/fitres_FAQ.html

This document contains information about exercise and fitness equipment and clothing for fat people. The makers of this page describe it as a source of information for the fat folks who do want to exercise.

Fitness World

http://www.fitnessworld.com/

In addition to current issues of the magazine, this site provides information about exercise books and videos, recent news highlights related to health and fitness, and answers to frequently asked questions about fitness. For fitness professionals, it also provides business information and opportunities to exchange with fellow professionals.

part

2

The Kinesiology Worldwide Home Page

http://www.umich.edu/~divkines/kinesworld/

A jumpsite to many kinesiology-related Web sites around the world.

National Athletic Trainers' Association

http://www.nata.org/

The National Athletic Trainers' Association (NATA) is a not-for-profit organization dedicated to improving the health and well-being of athletes worldwide. The Association is committed to the advancement, encouragement, and improvement of the athletic training profession.

National Coalition for Promoting Physical Activity

http://www.ncppa.org/

This is a premier organization in the country to promote physical activity. The objective of NCPPA is to unite the strengths of public, private and industry efforts into a collaborative partnership to inspire Americans to lead physically active lifestyles to enhance their health and quality of life.

New Zealand Fitness Home Page

http://home.ait.ac.nz/staff/pmellow//

Outstanding resource to links and information on fitness, sports, and health through exercise.

The Physician and Sports Medicine Online

http://www.physsportsmed.com/

This Web site features abstracts from the current issue of the magazine, actual articles from previous issues, a search feature to find selected topics from back issues, and a Personal Health section with patient-oriented articles on exercise, nutrition, and injury prevention.

Road Runners Club of America

http://rrca.org/

Novice and experienced runners alike will find a vast array of information provided by this not-for-profit organization, including a calendar of events, guidelines for putting on a race, how to start a club, and tips for running safely.

The Running Page

`http://sunsite.unc.edu/drears/running/running.html`

The Running Page contains information about upcoming races, race results, places to run, running related products, magazines, and other information.

Runner's World Online

`http://www.runnersworld.com/`

This site contains a wide variety of information about running, including tips for beginning runners, advice about training, and a shoe buyer's guide.

Selected Fitness, Exercise, Nutrition, Food, and Low Fat Recipe Sources

`http://www.idbsu.edu/carol/wellness.htm`

Numerous resources and links to information on many health related topics including those listed in the title.

WWW Women's Sports Page

`http://fiat.gslis.utexas.edu/~lewisa/womsprt.html`

An excellent jumpsite to women's sports pages around the WWW. Some of the topics include womens sports, womens sports organizations, and issues in womens sports.

WorldGuide Health and Fitness Forum

`http://www.worldguide.com/Fitness/hf.html`

Information on anatomy, strength training, cardiovascular exercise, eating well, sports medicine, etc.

part
2

General Health

Clearinghouse—Health and Medicine

http://www.clearinghouse.net/cgi-bin/chadmin/viewcat/
Health___Medicine?kywd++

This page is an enormous resource of a very wide range of health topics. Choose one and then click the hypertext link to up-to-date information.

Duke University Healthy Devil: On-line

http://h-devil-www.mc.duke.edu/h-devil

A general health resource location from Duke University. Contains a large list of health topics with basic definitions.

Fitlife

http://www.fitlife.com/

This resource provides current scientific information and services for four main areas of interest: wellness, fitness, current topics, and reader services.

Galaxy-Health

http://galaxy.einet.net/galaxy/Community/Health.html

This Web site is a galaxy search for community health topics and links.

Go Ask Alice

http://www.cc.columbia.edu:80/cu/healthwise/

Interactive answers to questions on various health topics.

Hardin Meta Directory for Internet Health Information

http://www.arcade.uiowa.edu/hardin-www/md.html

Pointers to the most complete and frequently cited lists in many health subject—a bit more medically oriented, but good.

part 2

Healthtouch

http://www.healthtouch.com/

Information on dozens of health topics and diseases as well as a medication guide on drug uses, precautions, and side effects.

Health World Online

http://www.healthy.net/

Provides 10 categories of health and wellness topics for consumers and professionals including nutrition, mind-body connection, and a medical library.

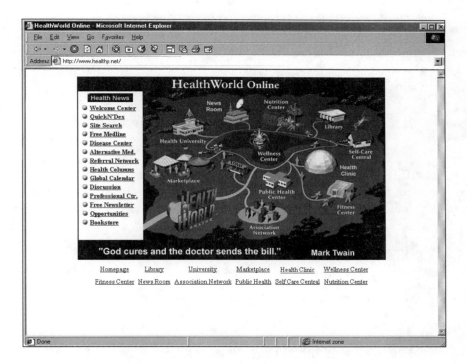

KidsHealth

http://www.kidshealth.org/index2.html

A mighty Web site devoted to the health of children and teens. Created by the medical experts at the Nemours Foundation, KidsHealth has trainloads of accurate, up-to-date information about growth, food, fitness, childhood infections, immunizations, lab tests, medical and surgical conditions, and the latest treatments. You'll find health games, How The Body Works animations, the KidsVote health poll, and tons of surprises. So get on board and explore!

The Longevity Game

http://www.northwesternmutual.com/games/longevity/

See how old you'll be before you pass on.

Mediconsult.com, Inc.

http://www.mediconsult.com/

This health Web site is one of the most complete and comprehensive health and medical info pages on the net. It gathers up-to-date information on all topics of health from journal reviews to the latest news. This is a great Web site. Spend some time here and you will be amazed.

National Council Against Health Fraud, Inc. (NCAHF)

http://www.ncahf.org/

These folks are the health information watchdogs. NCAHF is a non-profit, tax-exempt, voluntary health agency that focuses its attention upon health fraud, misinformation, and quackery as public health problems.

U.S. Healthcare Healthwatch

http://www.aetnaushc.com/topics/index.html

Good informational resource on many health topics. Includes a search index.

The Wellness Interactive Network

http://www.stayhealthy.com/

Self-described as a Web site with access to thousands of health information resources on the Internet.

Yahoo! Health Search Results

http://www.yahoo.com/Health

Contains links to health sites of all types, shapes, and sizes.

You First

http://www.youfirst.com/

This is a highly personalized, confidential, and interactive opportunity to determine your health risks with free online health risk appraisal. The Web site includes links to seasonal health tips, America's health risks, top 10 causes of death, and answers to frequently asked questions.

Health and Disease Care

AMSO Managed Care Forum

part
2

http://www.amso.com

The purpose the AMSO Web page is to provide a forum for the health-care professional and consumers of healthcare to learn and expound about the ever-changing managed healthcare industry.

CenterWatch Clinical Trials Listing Service

http://www.centerwatch.com/

You can use this listing to search for clinical trials, find out information about physicians and medical centers performing clinical research, and to learn about drug therapies newly approved by the Food and Drug Administration.

Convergent Medical Systems

http://www.convergentmedical.com/

This site has information relating to: healthcare consultants, strategic, managed care, health policy planning, health insurance, medical education, medical regulation, health promotion, wellness programs, allied health professions, alternative and complementary medicine, and world medicine.

GlobalMedic

http://www.globalmedic.com/

Empowering healthcare users through education and prevention. This interesting site includes a Medical Encyclopedia, nutrition information, and health information for women and children.

Health Care Liability Alliance

http://www.wp.com/HCLA/

A national advocacy coalition that supports effective federal health care liability reform to enhance the fairness, timeliness and cost-effectiveness of the civil justice system in resolving health care injury disputes.

Idea Central—Health Policy

http://epn.org/idea/health.html

A virtual magazine of the Electronic Policy Network. Offers information on HMOs, Medicaid, and other health policy issues. Updated monthly.

LIFE: Life and Health Insurance Information Site

http://www.life-line.org/index2.html

An excellent educational site designed to provide you with straightforward, unbiased information on life and health insurance.

Yahoo! Internet Search—Health Care

http://www.yahoo.com/Health/Health_Care/

This is a full Internet search of all things related to health care using the Yahoo! search engine.

School Health Education

American Cancer Society—Comprehensive School Health

http://www.cancer.org/cshe/cshe.html

Excellent resource for information on school health education.

ERIC Clearinghouse on Teaching and Teacher Education

http://www.ericsp.org/

A great site for information and Internet resources for education, teachers, teachers organizations, publications, financial aid, professional development schools, educational materials and resources, and more.

ERIC Clearinghouse on Teaching and Teacher Education: Health, Physical Education, Recreation, and Dance Divisions

http://www.ericsp.org/hprdtoc.html

ERIC's home page (see previous listing) in specialty areas listed in title.

The Health Education Hitlist

http://www.ex.ac.uk/~dregis/healthy.html

A jumpsite to World Wide Web pages for those interested in health education including, indices and search engines, school health resource services, health education, health care, public health, and other health issues.

Health Education Professional Resources (HEPR)

http://www.nyu.edu/education/hepr/

Extensive resource site for Health Education Professionals.

Health Promotion

Association for Worksite Health Promotion

http://www.awhp.com/

AWHP is a not-for-profit network of worksite health promotion professionals dedicated to sharing the best-of-practice methods, processes, and technologies. Site includes information on AWHP as well as other resources and links to wellness, health, and fitness pages.

Institue of Health Promotion Research

http://www.ihpr.ubc.ca/

Their mission is to provide a UBC focus for interdisciplinary collaboration on research, education, and community partnerships in health promotion.

Monash Health Promotion on the Internet

http://www.monash.edu.au/health/

Australia's Monash University's page on health promotion. It features a health promotion interactive lounge, and information and sites for the following: patient education, calendar of health events, Internet health directory, health resources, and health promotion research and education.

Rural Health Resources

http://www.siu.edu/~crhssd/rhres.htm

SIU center for Rural Health and Social Service Development. An excellent site with information and links to many great resources including, rural health resources, health agencies, medical resources, publications, socioeconomic data resources, search engines, and Web page and HTML help guides.

WellTech International

http://www.welltech.com/

One of the best resources for information and links for health promotion and wellness professionals.

Health Psychology

Alcoholics Anonymous Resources: A Collection of AA Information

http://www.recovery.org/aa/

Information and links on many aspects of AA including literature, history, intergroup phone numbers, meetings, conventions, computer programs, and links to more AA related resources.

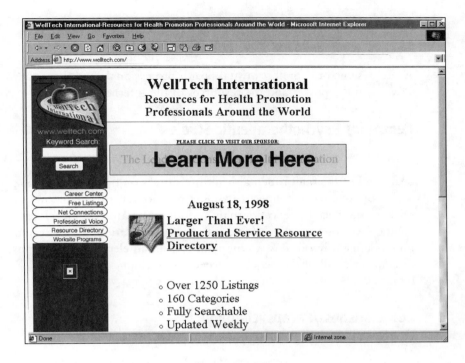

American Psychological Association

http://www.apa.org/

This is the home page of the APA. It includes the newspaper of the American Psychological Association, as well as other links and information to books, journals, employment, public practice, education information, and much more.

As a Man Thinketh

http://www.concentric.net/~conure/allen.html

The entire text of this fantastic little book online.

Astromind

http://www.astromind.is/index.html

This page is filled with exercises and ideas for increasing one's mental and spiritual powers.

At Health Inc.

http://www.athealth.com/

A site designed to connect mental health professionals and those they serve with the power and the resources of the Internet.

Centre for Psychotherapeutic Studies

http://www.shef.ac.uk/~psysc/psychotherapy/index.html

Search all of the major mental health resources on the World Wide Web from one page; connect to all 857 psychology, psychiatry, neuroscience, and social science journals and journal search engines; locate mental health texts, search for a colleague, a quotation, an electronic book, define a word, find a synonym, consult an electronic biography, or connect to all of the major Internet search engines. This site is remarkable!

Consciousness/Parapsychology/ Transpersonal Psychology

http://www.uwsp.edu/acad/psych/dk/danielpg.htm

This is a very interesting page by a professor at University of Wisconsin–Stevens Point. His emphases and the links on this page are devoted to consciousness, altered states of consciousness, parapsychology, and transpersonal psychology.

Dr. John Grohol's Mental Health Page

http://www.coil.com/~grohol/

This site is in the top 5% of all Web sites. A very good psychological resource site for psychology, support, and mental health issues, resources, and people.

Infinity Institute International

http://www.infinityinst.com/

An excellent resource on hypnosis and self-hypnosis.

Magic Stream

http://fly.hiwaay.net/~garson/

Journal of Emotional Wellness. The Web Dex contains extensive links on topics such as: addictions, recovery, child abuse, fitness, nutrition, depression, family, etc. The Journal contains original poetry, essays, articles, and short stories focused on personal growth and the universal in human emotion.

MedWeb: Mental Health, Psychiatry, Psychology

http://www.gen.emory.edu/MEDWEB/keyword/
mental_health~psychiatry~psychology.html

Excellent and extensive sites and resources for many aspects of mental health information.

Mental Health Net

http://www.cmhc.com/

A comprehensive guide to mental health online, featuring over 7,000 resources. Site has information on disorders such as depression, anxiety, panic attacks, chronic fatigue syndrome, substance abuse, professional resources in psychology, psychiatry and social work, journals, and self-help magazines.

Pie Online

http://pie.org/E18634T3783

Top mental and health Web sites for associations, foundations, government, health publications, mental health, public policy, research institutes, Web gateways, cool sites, search the Net links, and Pie home page.

Psychology Links

http://www.psyunix.iupui.edu/psych_dir.html

Links to organizations, journals, departments, and other resources having to do with psychology.

part
2

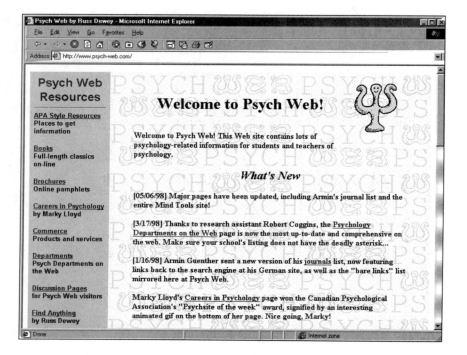

Psychology Self-Help Resources on the Internet

http://www.psych-web.com/

This page contains links to non-commercial sites providing information and help about specific disorders related to psychology. Excellent and extensive resources.

Sleep Medicine Home Page

http://www.cloud9.net/~thorpy/

This home page lists resources regarding all aspects of sleep including, the physiology of sleep, clinical sleep medicine, sleep research, federal and state information, patient information, and business-related groups.

Spiritual Consciousness

http://www.nerdworld.com/users/dstein/nw142.html

This is an enormous resource of spiritual health related Web sites around the world.

The Taoism Information Page

http://www.clas.ufl.edu/users/gthursby/taoism/

This page contains almost everything relevant to the philosophy of Taoism.

Zen Stories to Tell Your Neighbors

http://www1.rider.edu/~suler/zenstory/zenstory.html

This is a very nice collection of thought provoking Zen stories. Zensational!

Heart Health

American Heart Association

http://www.americanheart.org/

part
2

This site provides information on hundreds of topics relating to cardio-vascular health and disease, including cardiorespiratory endurance exercise.

Can Heart Disease Really Be Prevented?

http://www.cardio.com/articles/preventn.htm

By Peter M. Abel M.D., Medical Director, Prevention Center for Cardiovascular Disease Cardiovascular Institute of the South/Morgan City. Excellent information and sites to many other resources on heart disease.

Cardiovascular Institute of the South

http://www.cardio.com/

CIS, a leading center for the advanced diagnosis and treatment of heart and circulatory disease, presents a wide-ranging library of doctor column-style reports on this vital and rapidly evolving aspect of medi-cine.These reports cover the full spectrum of prevention, diagnosis, and nonsurgical and surgical treatment of circulatory problems.

Franklin Science Institute

http://www.fi.edu/biosci/heart.html

This site provides learning opportunities about how the heart functions in an interactive lab simulation. This is a very interesting Web site on the heart.

Healthy Heart

http://sln.fi.edu/biosci/healthy/healthy.html

Excellent information on a wide range of subjects pertaining to a healthy heart including educational and enrichment activities.

Late Breaking News for Heart Health

http://www.mindspring.com/~mtm/news.html

part
2

This site is dedicated to natural health, alternative medicine, and the latest available news related to the improvement of overall health of men and women over 35.

Linus C. Pauling

http://www.Internetwks.com/pauling/

This is an interesting webpage on reversing heart disease without surgury (extensive info-site). It follows much of the theories and ideas espoused by the late Linus Pauling.

The Learning Center

http://www.hsforum.com/HeartSurgery/
LearningCtrHSF.html

Heart Disease and your health—what you should know. This page provides information and explanations of common cardiovascular diseases specifically for the non-medical audience.

Vegetarian Diets

http://www.fatfree.com/FAQ/ada-paper

This page contains a position paper by the American Dietetic Association. It states the Association's summary of the healthful nature of a vegetarian diet.

Food and Nutrition

American Dietetics Association Homepage

http://www.eatright.org/

A Web page designed to promote optimal nutrition, health, and well-being. Contains nutrition information and resources.

The American Heart Association Diet

http://www.amhrt.org/catalog/Health_catpage4.html

This eating plan from the American Heart Association describes the latest advice of medical and nutritional experts. The best way to help lower your blood cholesterol is to eat less saturated fatty acids and cholesterol and control your weight. The AHA Diet gives you an easy-to-follow guide to eating with your heart in mind.

Arbor Communications Nutrition Resources on the Internet

http://arborcom.com/

This site contains one of the most comprehensive lists available of Internet nutrition resources.

Arizona Health Sciences Library Nutrition Guide

http://www.medlib.arizona.edu/educ/nutrition.html

This is an extremely comprehensive page on most aspects of nutrition from the University of Arizona.

Ask the Dietition

http://www.dietitian.com/

This is a question and answer page on nearly all aspects of nutrition.

Aspartame (Nutrasweet) Toxicity Information Center

http://www.holisticmed.com/aspartame/

Detailed scientific and general documentation regarding the toxicity of Nutrasweet, Equal, Diet Coke, Diet Pepsi, and other aspartame-

part

2

containing items. Web page includes real life reports of acute and chronic toxicity due to long-term ingestion. Also included is extensive scientific and general information and resources.

Diet and Weight Loss/Fitness Home Page

http://www1.mhv.net/~donn/diet.html

Great site offering FAQs about dieting, weight loss tips from readers, weight tables comparison study, news wire summaries, all about calories, and multiple links to Ask the Dietitian, Artificial Sweetener Controversy, Vegetarians, and many others. There are also links to fitness sites and information on support groups.

Electronic Gourmet Guide

http://www.foodwine.com/

This is a very tantalizing page with a lot of interesting information on food.

Fast Food Facts—Interactive Food Finder

http://www.olen.com/food/

This is a wonderful page designed to help anyone determine the ingredients of his or her favorite fast foods. Very interactive and useful. This is one of my personal favorites.

Food and Nutrition: Selected Electronic Resources

http://www.nalusda.gov/fnic/

This is an excellent Web site that may be the first place to search for anything related to food and nutrition.

The Food Pyramid

http://www.ganesa.com/food/index.html

Up-to-date information on the latest information on what we used to know as the four food groups.

part
2

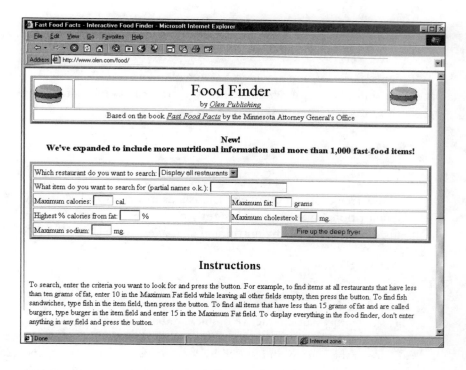

Health and Nutrition

http://dinnercoop.cs.cmu.edu/dinnercoop/special/
health.html

This is a page filled with nothing but more links to nutrition information around the world. It contains a very large number of links.

Human Health and Nutrition

http://www.envirolink.org/arrs/health_wrap.html

Animal rights resource site. Contains information and links on nutrition and health that follow their philosophies.

International Food Information Council

http://ificinfo.health.org/

This page is designed to enhance consumers' abilities to make informed food choices by developing and supporting informational and educational programs on food safety, nutrition and health. Includes a lot of good information relating to healthy hearts.

part

2

Mother Nature's General Store

http://www.mothernature.com/

Forums, libraries, and resources on nutrition and food. This page includes information on vitamins, herbs, recipes, and other interesting health information. Outstanding Web site.

My Menus

http://www.mymenus.com/

The best recipe site on the Web! Thousands of nutritional recipes. Complete nutritional information. Instantly custom-build your own meal plans. Look up recipes by nutritional characteristic. YUMMY STUFF!

Nutribase On-Line

http://www.nutribase.com/

This site features an interactive online database of over 19,000 food items and their associated nutrient information . . . food items that you can view, rank, query, and search by food names. This database includes more than 3,000 menu items from over 70 restaurants. This site also features a weight-loss calculator, a calorie requirements calculator, desirable weight and body fat content charts, a directory of 1,400 food and supplement makers, a listing of healthy food substitutions, a glossary of foods and cooking terms, toll-free numbers for food makers, and 1,000 quotes and tips for dieters. It's all here!

Veggies Unite!

http://www.vegweb.com/

This is a central site for all things vegetarian.

Public Health

APHA

http://www.apha.org/

Home page for the American Public Health Association.

part
2

Career Espresso!

http://www.sph.emory.edu/studentservice/Career.html

The absolute hottest public health career search Web site anywhere!

CDC

http://www.cdc.gov/

Home page for the Center for Disease Control.

The Virtual Public Health Center

http://www-sci.lib.uci.edu/~martindale/PHealth.html

Possibly the most comprehensive resource out there on public health.

Safety and Injury Prevention

Bicycle Helmet Safety Institute

http://www.bhsi.org/index.htm

This is a small, active, non-profit consumer-funded program acting as a clearinghouse and a technical resource for bicycle helmet information. Includes information on statistics, publications, laws, and advice on bicycle helmet safety as well as other helmet and bicycle type links.

Christie's Safety Related Internet Resources

http://www.mrg.ab.ca/christie/safelist.htm

Christie Communication services safety associations, large and small business, formal educational institutions, and government with educational information and training materials.

Consumer Product Safety Commission

gopher://cpsc.gov/

The U.S. Consumer Product Safety Commission (CPSC), is an independent federal regulatory agency that was created in 1972 by Congress in the Consumer Product Safety Act. This page is a gopher server that contains lots of information and links regarding consumer product safety.

National Safety Council

http://www.nsc.org/

National Safety Council's mission is to educate and influence society to adopt safety, health, and environmental policies, practices, and procedures that prevent and mitigate human suffering and economic losses arising from preventable causes.

Product Safety Link Directory

http://www.safetylink.com/

This site has extensive information and links to many aspects of product safety.

part

2

Poisons Information Database

http://vhp.nus.sg/PID/

Information on natural toxins and poisons, and directories of antivenoms, toxinologists, and poison control centers around the world.

Public Health and Safety

http://www.yahoo.com/Health/Public_Health_And_Safety/

Yahoo! references to public health and safety issues include, disasters, EMF health issues, fire protection, flouridation, helmets, institutions, law enforcement, lead poisoning, lifesaving/lifeguarding, magazines, organizations, safety products, and much more.

U.S. Environmental Protection Agency

http://www.epa.gov/

This site contains a wealth of information about the agency and environmental issues as well as links to many other environmental and safety resources.

Self-Help and Self-Care

Cal Berkeley Wellness Letter

http://www.enews.com/magazines/ucbwl/

The Wellness Letter is edited by research scientists and written in lay English. Features the latest news from the world of preventive medicine and practical advice on all aspects of healthy living.

Healthfinder

http://www.healthfinder.org/default.htm

Healthfinder is a gateway consumer health information Web site from the United States government. Healthfinder can lead you to selected on-line publications, databases, Web sites, and support and self-help groups, as well as the government agencies and not-for-profit organizations that produce reliable health information for the public.

The Life Extension Foundation

http://www.lef.org/

The Life Extension Foundation is dedicated to the pursuit of a longer, healthier lifespan. We provide our members with information about the latest life extension research, products, and therapies.

LifeMatters

http://lifematters.com/index.html

A very interesting site that describes itself as an ongoing conversation about taking charge of one's health and well-being for a life that is empowered, fulfilled, and profoundly related.

The Other Revolution in Health Care

http://www.hotwired.com/wired/2.01/features/
healthcare.html

This site contains an interesting article on health care.

part
2

Personal Development Central

http://www.ns.net/~sjmoore/psites.html

Links to many journals, organizations, networks, businesses, and other information sources dealing with personal development.

Psychology Self-Help Resources on the Internet

http://www.gasou.edu/psychweb/resource/selfhelp.htm

This site contains links to non-commercial sites providing information and help about specific disorders related to psychology. Excellent and extensive resources.

Self-Help

http://www.lib.ox.ac.uk/Internet/news/faq/archive/
self-impr-faq.part1.html

Frequently asked questions on currently popular self-help resources such as NLP, speed reading, hypnosis and many others. This is an excellent source of information on a huge list of topics.

Self-Help (pt. 2)

http://www.lib.ox.ac.uk/Internet/news/faq/archive/
self-impr-faq.part2.html

Part two of the previous Web site.

Self-Help Links Category Page

http://cybertowers.com/cgibin/
add_a_link.cgi?all_links=go

Click on one of the topics in this huge list and you will find a huge amount of related information.

Web Links for Medical and Mental Health Problems

http://www.realtime.net/~mmjw/

An excellent source for many resources and links in many areas of medical and mental health. This site has been rated in the top 5 percent of all Web sites.

part

2

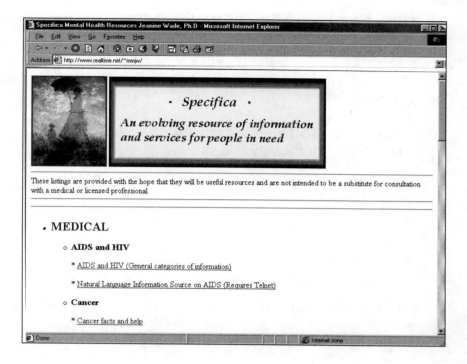

Stress Management

The American Institute of Stress

http://www.stress.org/index.htm

The home page for the the institute that is dedicated to advancing our knowledge of the role of stress in health and disease.

The Anxiety-Panic Internet Resource

http://www.algy.com/anxiety/anxiety.html

This page gathers information of interest to those with the characteristic symptoms of debilitating anxiety, panic attacks, phobias, obsessive thoughts, and/or depression.

How to Fight and Conquer Stress

http://www.coolware.com/health/joel/stress.html

This is an information page on stress as it affects us and some ideas on how to deal with it.

Introduction to Stress Management, NLP, and Hypnotherapy

http://www.bogo.co.uk/andys/index.html

This page includes a link to more good information on managing stress before it manages you.

Relax.calm

http://www.concord.wvnet.edu/~olpin/relax.html

This page is designed to give you resources that can help you manage your stress more effectively. It contains excellent links, great resources, and some valuable tips and guidelines that will certainly appeal to you as you are trying to find a healthy balance in these stressful times.

StressFreeNET

http://www.stressfree.com/

StressFree Network is a system of health care professionals providing solutions to stress. They provide confidential assistance to individuals, business, and occupational groups for whom stress is an important issue.

The Web's Stress Management and Emotional Wellness Page

http://imt.net/~randolfi/StressPage.html

This is a great resource for stress management including some excellent links and ideas for managing stress.

Tobacco, Alcohol, and Drug Use

AIRSPACE Non-smokers' Rights Society

http://www.seercom.com/airspace/

AIRSPACE's goals are to require all indoor public places be smoke-free, to prohibit the sale of tobacco to minors, to prohibit all forms of tobacco promotion, and to hold the tobacco industry accountable for the disease and death caused by their product.

Al-Anon and Alateen

http://www.Al-Anon-Alateen.org/

AL-ANON (and ALATEEN for younger members) is a worldwide organization that offers a self-help recovery program for families and friends of alcoholics whether or not the alcoholic seeks help or even recognizes the existence of a drinking problem.

Center for Alcohol and Addiction Studies

http://center.butler.brown.edu/

Located at Brown University, the Center's mission is to promote the identification, prevention and effective treatment of alcohol and other drug use problems in our society through research, publications, education, and training.

Drug-Related Network Resources

http://hyperreal.com/drugs/faqs/resources.html

This is a large list of links to many sites related to drugs of all types. Includes information on both sides of the controversies surrounding drugs.

Join Together Online

http://www.jointogether.org/jto/

Homepage of a national resource center and meeting place for communities working to reduce substance abuse (illicit drugs, excessive alcohol, tobacco) and gun violence.

part

2

National Clearinghouse for Alcohol and Drug Information

http://www.health.org/aboutn.htm

This is the information service of the Center for Substance Abuse Prevention of the U.S. Department of Health and Human Services. NCADI is the world's largest resource for current information and materials concerning substance abuse prevention.

National Institute on Drug Abuse

http://www.nida.nih.gov/

This Web site with information on the NIDA includes its organizations, calendar of events, communications, grants, and links to other related web sites.

National Inhalant Prevention Coalition

http://www.inhalants.com/

This is a very comprehensive page devoted to disseminating accurate information about inhalants.

part 2

National Women's Resource Center

http://www.nwre.org/

This page provides information on prevention of alcohol, tobacco, and drug abuse.

The Nicotine and Tobacco Network

http://tobacco.arizona.edu/

Great resource from the University of Arizona. Contains links and information on research, news, programs, resources, and other items relating to nicotine and tobacco.

Prevline: Prevention Hotline and National Clearinghouse for Alcohol and Drugs

http://www.health.org/

This site provides a comprehensive database of alcohol and drug information and links.

Smoking from All Sides

http://www.cs.brown.edu/people/lsh/smoking.html

Links to Web sites on many aspects of smoking including, health aspects, statistics, tobacco news, anti-smoking groups, smoking cessation, tobacco history, commentary, pro-smoking documents, smoking glamour, etc.

Tobacco BBS

http://www.tobacco.org/

This is a resource center focusing on tobacco and smoking issues. It features tobacco news and information, assistance for smokers trying to quit, as well as a wide spectrum of tobacco-related concerns. It also offers a unique list of links to tobacco-related art, books, films, and anti-smoking activism.

Violence Resources and Information

part **2**

Domestic Violence in the Workplace

http://www.igc.apc.org/fund/workplace/

A Web site with articles, information, and sites to many aspects of domestic violence.

Domestic Violence: The Facts

http://www.igc.apc.org/fund/the_facts/

A Web site with facts, information, and links to other sources dealing with domestic violence.

National Crisis Prevention Institute's Violence Prevention Resource Center

http://www.execpc.com/~cpi/

CPI offers training in the safe management of disruptive and assaultive behavior, as well as other topics in areas such as business, mental health, corrections, security, police, youth and human services, and government.

National Institute for Occupational Safety and Health (NIOSH)

http://www.cdc.gov/niosh/homepage.html

NIOSH is a federal agency established by the Occupational Safety and Health Act of 1970. NIOSH is part of the Centers for Disease Control and Prevention (CDC) and is responsible for conducting research and making recommendations for the prevention of work-related illness and injuries.

OSHA Guidelines for Workplace Violence Prevention Programs

http://www.osha-slc.gov/OshDoc/Additional.html

This site contains several articles relating to worksite violence.

The Rockem-Sockem Workplace

http://venable.com/wlu/rockem.htm

This is an informative article on violence in the workplace.

part

2

Weight Control

Ask the Dietitian/Overweight

http://www.dietitian.com/overweig.html

This is an excellent question and answer page relating to weight control, nutrition, and activity.

Cyberdiet

http://www.cyberdiet.com/

This site includes assessments tools, an online nutritional profile, a daily food planner, a database of foods, recipe index, and more.

Diet and Weight Loss/Fitness Home Page

http://www1.mhv.net/~donn/diet.html

Great site offering FAQs about dieting, weight loss tips from readers, weight tables comparison study, news wire summaries, all about calories, and multiple links to Ask the Dietitian, Artificial Sweetener Controversy,

Vegetarians, and many others. There are also links to fitness sites and information on support groups.

Healthy Weight

http://healthyweight.com/

This Web site provides consumers, health care professionals and the media with valuable resources for weight management and healthy living. It contains related news, links, and a newsletter. An excellent resource.

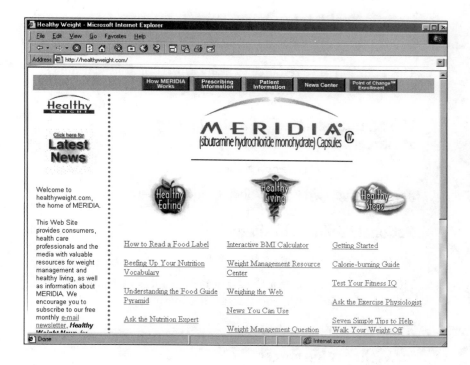

part

2

Shape Up America

http://www2.shapeup.org/sua/index.html

This Web site is designed to provide you with the latest information about safe weight management and physical fitness.

What is Obesity?

http://www.weight.com/comprehensive.html

This page contains a discussion on how to lose weight permanently.

Wellness and Optimum Health

HealthWise Newsletter

http://www.columbia.edu/cu/healthwise/

The Health Education and Wellness program of Columbia University Health Service.

Holistic Health Information Page

http://www.tiac.net/users/mgold/health.html

This is an extensive resource to many aspects of holistic healing and health.

The Mind/Body Medical Institute at Harvard Medical School

http://www.med.harvard.edu/programs/mindbody/

Resource page to the Mind/Body Clinic. Extensive information.

National Wellness Institute

http://www.wellnessnwi.org/

This is the home page for the National Wellness Institute, including the departments and conferences associated with it.

Wellness Community Center—A Magnet for Wellness Resources

http://www.aboutliving.com/htmlal/index.html

The Wellness Directory is a central reference tool to help Internet users find resources relating to spirituality, emotional growth, and mental development. The Directory provides listings and links within the categories of: For Parents, For Kids, Spirit & Myth, Art, Music, Poetry, Search Engines, Directories, and In the Workplace.

The Whole Balance Catalogue

http://hyperlink.com/balance

A monthly publication devoted mainly to higher levels of health and well-being with articles devoted to these topics.

Women's Health

Altanta Reproductive Health Centre

http://www.ivf.com/

Excellent resources for topics of interest to women. One of the best out there.

Breastfeeding Articles and Resources

http://www.parentsplace.com/readroom/bf.html

This page includes articles and information on nearly every question anyone could ever ask regarding breastfeeding.

MedWeb Gynecology and women's health

http://www.gen.emory.edu/medweb/medweb.gynecology.html

Excellent resource with extensive links for a great number of women's medical and health issues.

Melpomene Institute for Women's Health Research

http://www.melpomene.org/

This not-for-profit Minneapolis based institute, named for the first female marathon runner, specializes in health issues affecting physically active women. This Web site features topics geared to active girls and women of all ages, such as exercise during pregnancy, body image, osteoporosis, and menopause.

Natural Progesterone and Women's Health

http://www.health-science.com/health.htm

This is a page with information on PMS, fertility, menopause, osteoporosis, and other women's health topics.

Sexual Assault Information

http://www.cs.utk.edu/~bartley/saInfoPage.html

This page includes a nice search for many subtopics falling under the main topic of sexual assault. This is an excellent reference.

Women's' Health America Group

http://www1.fourlakes.net/~wha/

Dynamic national organization whose mission is to encourage and enable women to make informed decisions about their healthcare by providing access to current and accurate information and quality health products.

Women's Health Information

http://www.yahoo.com/Health/Women_s_Health/

This is a Yahoo! search for all things on the Internet related to Women's Health.

Documentation

 ## Your Citation for Exemplary Research

There's another detail left for us to handle—the formal citing of electronic sources in academic papers. The very factor that makes research on the Internet exciting is the same factor that makes referencing these sources challenging: their dynamic nature. A journal article exists, either

part
2

in print or on microfilm, virtually forever. A document on the Internet can come, go, and change without warning. Because the purpose of citing sources is to allow another scholar to retrace your argument, a good citation allows a reader to obtain information from your primary sources, to the extent possible. This means you need to include not only information on when a source was posted on the Internet (if available) but also when you obtained the information.

The two arbiters of form for academic and scholarly writing are the Modern Language Association (MLA) and the American Psychological Association (APA); both organizations have established styles for citing electronic publications.

MLA Style

In the second edition of the *MLA Style Manual,* the MLA recommends the following formats:

- URLs: URLs are enclosed in angle brackets (<>) and contain the access mode identifier, the formal name for such indicators as "http" or "ftp." If a URL must be split across two lines, break it only after a slash (/). Never introduce a hyphen at the end of the first line. The URL should include all the parts necessary to identify uniquely the file/document being cited.

    `<http://www.csun.edu/~rtvfdept/home/index.html>`

- A complete online reference contains the title of the project or database (underlined); the name of the editor of the project or database (if given); electronic publication information, including version number (if relevant and if not part of the title); date of electronic publication or latest update; name of any sponsoring institution or organization; date of access; and electronic address.

- If you cannot find some of the information, then include the information that is available.

The MLA also recommends that you print or download electronic documents, freezing them in time for future reference.

World Wide Web Site   The elements of a proper citation are the name of the person creating the site (reversed), followed by a period, the title of the site (underlined), or, if there is no title, a description such as home page (such a description is neither placed in quotes nor underlined).

part **2**

Then specify the name of any school, organization, or other institution affiliated with the site and follow it with your date of access and the URL of the page.

Gotthoffer, Doug. <u>RTVF Dept. Website</u>. California
State University, Northridge. 1 September 1998.

Some electronic references are truly unique to the online domain. These include email, newsgroup postings, MUDs (multiuser domains) or MOOs (multiuser domains, object oriented), and IRCs (Internet Relay Chats).

Email   In citing email messages, begin with the writer's name (reversed) followed by a period, then the title of the message (if any) in quotations as it appears in the subject line. Next comes a description of the message, typically "Email to," and the recipient (e.g., "the author"), and finally the date of the message.

Davis, Jeffrey. "Web Writing Resources." Email to
Nora Davis. 5 July 1998.

Sommers, Laurice. "Re: College Admissions Practices."
Email to the author. 12 August 1998.

List Servers and Newsgroups   In citing these references, begin with the author's name (reversed) followed by a period. Next include the title of the document (in quotes) from the subject line, followed by the words "Online posting" (not in quotes). Follow this with the date of posting. For list servers, include the date of access, the name of the list (if known), and the online address of the list's moderator or administrator. For newsgroups, follow "Online posting" with the date of posting, the date of access, and the name of the newsgroup, prefixed with news: and enclosed in angle brackets.

Applebaum, Dale. "Educational Variables." Online
posting. 29 Jan. 1998. Higher Education
Discussion Group. 30 January 1993
<jlucidoj@unc.edu>.

Gostl, Jack. "Re: Mr. Levitan." Online posting.
13 June 1997. 20 June 1997
<news:alt.edu.bronxscience>.

MUDs, MOOs, and IRCs   Citations for these online sources take the form of the name of the speaker(s) followed by a period. Then comes the description and date of the event, the name of the forum, the date of access, and the online address prefixed by "telnet://".

```
Guest. Personal interview. 13 August 1998
    <telnet//du.edu 8888>.
```

APA Style

The *Publication Manual of the American Psychological Association* (4th ed.) is fairly dated in its handling of online sources, having been published before the rise of the WWW and the generally recognized format for URLs. The format that follows is based on the APA manual, with modifications proposed by Russ Dewey <www.psychwww.com/resource/apacrib.htm>. It's important to remember that, unlike the MLA, the APA does not include temporary or transient sources (e.g., letters, phone calls, etc.) in its "References" page, preferring to handle them in in-text citations exclusively. This rule holds for electronic sources as well: email, MOOs/MUDs, list server postings, etc., are not included in the "References" page, merely cited in text, for example, "But Wilson has rescinded his earlier support for these policies" (Charles Wilson, personal email to the author, 20 November 1996). But also note that many list server and Usenet groups and MOOs actually archive their correspondences, so that there is a permanent site (usually a Gopher or FTP server) where those documents reside. In that case, you would want to find the archive and cite it as an unchanging source. Strictly speaking, according to the APA manual, a file from an FTP site should be referenced as follows:

```
Deutsch, P. (1991). "Archie-An electronic directory
    service for the Internet" [Online]. Available
    FTP: ftp.sura.net Directory: pub/archie/docs
    File: whatis.archie.
```

However, the increasing familiarity of Net users with the convention of a URL makes the prose description of how to find a file <"Available FTP: ftp.sura.net Directory: pub/archie/docs File: whatis.archie"> unnecessary. Simply specifying the URL should be enough.

So, with such a modification of the APA format, citations from the standard Internet sources would appear as follows.

part
2

FTP (File Transfer Protocol) Sites To cite files available for downloading via FTP, give the author's name (if known), the publication date (if available and if different from the date accessed), the full title of the paper (capitalizing only the first word and proper nouns), the address of the FTP site along with the full path necessary to access the file, and the date of access.

```
Deutsch, P. (1991) "Archie-An electronic directory
    service for the Internet." [Online]. Available:
    ftp://ftp.sura.net/pub/archie/docs/whatis.archie.
```

WWW Sites (World Wide Web) To cite files available for viewing or downloading via the World Wide Web, give the author's name (if known), the year of publication (if known and if different from the date accessed), the full title of the article, and the title of the complete work (if applicable) in italics. Include any additional information (such as versions, editions, or revisions) in parentheses immediately following the title. Include the full URL (the http address) and the date of visit.

```
Burka, L. P. (1993). A hypertext history of multi-
    user dungeons. MUDdex. http://www.utopia.com/
    talent/lpb/muddex/essay/ (13 Jan. 1997).

Tilton, J. (1995). Composing good HTML (Vers. 2.0.6).
    http://www.cs.cmu.edu/~tilt/cgh/ (1 Dec. 1996).
```

Telnet Sites List the author's name or alias (if known), the date of publication (if available and if different from the date accessed), the title of the article, the title of the full work (if applicable) or the name of the Telnet site in italics, and the complete Telnet address, followed by a comma and directions to access the publication (if applicable). Last, give the date of visit in parentheses.

```
Dava (#472). (1995, 3 November). A deadline.
    *General (#554). Internet Public Library.
    telnet://ipl.sils.umich.edu:8888, @peek 25 on
    #554 (9 Aug. 1996).

Help. Internet public library.
    telnet://ipl.org:8888/, help (1 Dec. 1996).
```

Synchronous Communications (MOOs, MUDs, IRC, etc.) Give the name of the speaker(s), the complete date of the conversation being referenced in parentheses (if different from the date accessed), and the title of the session (if applicable). Next, list the title of the site in italics, the protocol and address (if applicable), and any directions necessary to access the work. If there is additional information such as archive addresses or file numbers (if applicable), list the word "Available," a colon, and the archival information. Last, list the date of access, enclosed in parentheses. Personal interviews do not need to be listed in the References, but do need to be included in parenthetic references in the text (see the APA *Publication Manual*).

Basic IRC commands. irc undernet.org, /help (13 Jan. 1996).

Cross, J. (1996, February 27). Netoric's Tuesday cafe: Why use MUDs in the writing classroom? MediaMoo. telenet://purple-crayon.media.mit.edu: 8888, @go Tuesday. Available: ftp://daedalus.com/ pub/ACW/NETORIC/catalog.96a (tc 022796.log). (1 Mar. 1996).

part
2

Gopher Sites List the author's name (if applicable), the year of publication (if known and if different from the date accessed), the title of the file or paper, and the title of the complete work (if applicable). Include any print publication information (if available) followed by the protocol (i.e., gopher://) and the path necessary to access the file. List the date that the file was accessed in parentheses immediately following the path.

Massachusetts Higher Education Coordinating Council. (1994) [Online]. Using coordination and collaboration to address change. Available: gopher://gopher.mass.edu:170/00gopher_root%3A%5B_ hecc%5D_plan.

Email, Listservs, and Newsgroups Give the author's name (if known), the date of the correspondence in parentheses (if known and if different from the date accessed), the subject line from the posting, and the name of the list (if known) in italics. Next, list the address of the listserv or newsgroup. Include any archival information after the address, listing the word "Available" and a colon and the protocol and address of the archive. Last, give the date accessed enclosed in parentheses. Do not include personal email in the list of References. See the APA *Publication Manual* for information on in-text citations.

Bruckman, A. S. MOOSE crossing proposal. mediamoo@media.mit.edu (20 Dec. 1994).

Heilke, J. (1996, May 3). Re: Webfolios. acw-l@ttacs. ttu.edu. Available: http://www.ttu.edu/lists/acw-l/ 9605 (31 Dec. 1996).

Laws, R. UMI thesis publication. alt.education. distance (3 Jan. 1996).

Other authors and educators have proposed similar extensions to the APA style, too. You can find URLs to these pages at

www.psychwww.com/resource/apacrib.htm

and

www.nouveaux.com/guides.htm

Another frequently-referenced set of extensions is available at

www.uvm.edu/~ncrane/estyles/apa.htm

Remember, "frequently-referenced" does not equate to "correct" or even "desirable." Check with your professor to see if your course or school has a preference for an extended APA style.

part
2

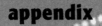

appendix

List of URLs
(Web Addresses)

Health News

```
http://www.achoo.com/features/headlinenews/index.htm
http://www.altmedicine.com/
http://www.eatright.org/pressindex.html
http://www.chronicillnet.org/online/
http://www.cnn.com/HEALTH/index.html
http://www.ljextra.com/practice/health/index.html
http://www.mayohealth.org/ivi/mayo/common/htm/newsstnd.htm
http://www.nando.net/nt/health/index_t.html
http://www.newspage.com/NEWSPAGE/cgi-bin/walk.cgi/
    NEWSPAGE/info/d15/
http://www.reutershealth.com/
http://www.newstimes.com/news/today/health.htm
http://www.usatoday.com/life/health/lhd1.htm
http://www.wellmedia.com/news.html
http://www.yahoo.com/headlines/health/
http://nytsyn.com/med/
```

Health Related Searches

```
http://www.altavista.digital.com/
http://www.webdirectory.com/Health/
http://my.excite.com/lifestyle/health_and_fitness/
http://www.einet.net/galaxy/Community/Health.html
http://www.HealthAtoZ.com/
http://guide-p.infoseek.com/Health?tid=1207
```

141

```
http://www.linkmonster.com/health.html
http://a2z.lycos.com/Health_and_Medicine/
http://www.mckinley.com/magellan/Reviews/
    Health_and_Medicine/index.magellan.html
http://www.medmatrix.org/index.asp
http://vh.radiology.uiowa.edu/Misc/Search.html
http://webcrawler.com/Health/
http://www.yahoo.com/Health/
```

Health Related Journals, Magazines, and Periodicals

```
http://www.allabouthealth.com/
http://www.forthrt.com/~chronicl/homepage.html
http://carlisle-www.army.mil/apfri/alive.htm
http://ww2.hyperlink.com/balance/
http://www.hinman.oro.net/~bmsweb/bmsmag.htm
http://primusweb.com/fitnesspartner/
http://www.lifelines.com/lifenews.html
http://healthnet.ivi.com/ivi/mayo/common/htm/library.htm
http://www.medscape.com/
http://mensfitness.com/
http://www.newfrontier.com/
http://www.newage.com/
http://www.nejm.org/
http://www.cspinet.org/nah/
http://pie.org/E21221T3783
http://www.physsportsmed.com/
http://www.well.com/user/selfhelp/index.html
http://www.shareguide.com/mag/
http://www.yogajournal.com/
```

appendix

Health Research and Evaluation

```
http://www.carl.org/Access.html
http://chid.nih.gov/
http://ericae.net/
http://www.healthfinder.gov/moretools/
http://weber.u.washington.edu/~hserv/authinst/jolist.html
http://www.healthgate.com/HealthGate/MEDLINE/search.shtml
http://www.homepage.holowww.com/
http://www.nyu.edu/education/hepr/resources/online/
    index.html
http://www.ovid.com/
http://www.cmhc.com/journals/
```

http://web.indstate.edu/hlthsfty/hlth341/home.htm
http://www.science.widener.edu/~withers/evalout.htm

Alternative Medicine and Holistic Health

http://www.Acupuncture.com/
http://www.pitt.edu/~cbw/altm.html
http://www.altmedicine.com/
http://www.rhemamed.com/altmed.htm
http://www.medicalmaze.com/index.html
http://healer.infinite.org/
http://www.amtamassage.org/
http://www.quake.net/~xdcrlab/hp.html
http://www.dreamup.com/
http://www.kcweb.com/herb/herbmain.htm
http://www.herbnet.com/
http://www.herbs.org/index.html
http://www.holisticmed.com/
http://www.homeopathyhome.com/
http://www.samart.co.th/hps/wwwresor.htm
http://login.samart.co.th/~hps/
http://www.nursery.com/~interlud/links.htm
http://www.iahf.com/
http://ezinfo.ucs.indiana.edu/~aeulenbe/i_see
http://www.gen.emory.edu/MEDWEB/keyword/
    alternative_medicine.html
http://www.teleport.com/~amrta/
http://altmed.od.nih.gov/
http://www.oxytherapy.com/
http://www.spiritweb.org/
http://ww2.hyperlink.com/weaver/
http://wellmedia.com/links.html

appendix

Cancer

http://www.cancer.org/
http://nysernet.org/bcic/
http://www.cancercareinc.org/
http://www.cancernews.com/
http://www.cansearch.org/canserch/canserch.htm
http://www.ncl.ac.uk/~nchwww/guides/clinks1.htm
http://africa.com/~martin/jomol/
http://www.nci.nih.gov/
http://cancernet.nci.nih.gov/pdq.htm

```
http://www.cancer.med.umich.edu/NCCN/NCCN.html
http://www.maui.net/~southsky/introto.html
http://cancerguide.org/
http://www.oncolink.upenn.edu/
http://www.yahoo.com/Health/Diseases_and_Conditions/Cancer/
```

Community Health Education

```
http://www.amhrt.org/
http://www.cdc.gov/cdc.html
http://web.indstate.edu/hlthsfty/ch/ch.htm
http://userwww.service.emory.edu/~cescoff/cam.html
http://nhic-nt.health.org/
http://www.nih.gov/
http://www.paho.org/
http://www.who.ch/
```

appendix

Diseases: Chronic and Acute

```
http://a2z.lycos.com/Health_and_Medicine/
    Illnesses_and_Disorders/
http://www.diabetes.org/
http://www.lungusa.org/
http://www.cdc.gov/diseases/diseases.html
http://www.chronicillnet.org/
http://www.mic.ki.se/Diseases/index.html
http://medhlp.netusa.net/
http://www.cdc.gov/epo/mmwr/mmwr.html
http://www.mothernature.com/hotlist.htm
http://ftp.cdc.gov/nccdphp/nccdhome.htm
http://www.sig.net/~allergy/welcome.html
http://point.lycos.com/topics/Conditions_Overall.html
http://med-www.bu.edu/people/sycamore/std/std.htm
http://www.bocklabs.wisc.edu/Welcome.html
http://www.yahoo.com/Health/Diseases_and_Conditions/
```

Environmental Health

```
http://atsdr1.atsdr.cdc.gov:8080/cx.html
http://www.cdc.gov/nceh/ncehhome.htm
http://www.niehs.nih.gov/
```

http://www.pacificrim.net/~nature/
http://www.yahoo.com/Health/Environmental_Health/

Exercise and Fitness

http://research.med.umkc.edu/aafp/Q19.html
http://www.aahperd.org/
http://www.a1.com/sportsmed/
http://www.acefitness.org/
http://www.cascade.org/links.html
http://www.clark.net/pub/pribut/spsport.html
http://members.aol.com/ironmaan/fitnesslab.html
http://www.sportlink.com/fitness/
http://www.noah.cuny.edu/pregnancy/march_of_dimes/
    pre_preg.plan/fit42is.html
http://www.comlab.ox.ac.uk/oucl/users/sharon.curtis/
    BigFolks/fitres_FAQ.html
http://www.fitnessworld.com/
http://www.umich.edu/~divkines/kinesworld/
http://www.nata.org/
http://www.ncppa.org/
http://home.ait.ac.nz/staff/pmellow//
http://www.physsportsmed.com/
http://rrca.org/
http://sunsite.unc.edu/drears/running/running.html
http://www.runnersworld.com/
http://www.idbsu.edu/carol/wellness.htm
http://fiat.gslis.utexas.edu/~lewisa/womsprt.html
http://www.worldguide.com/Fitness/hf.html

appendix

General Health

http://www.clearinghouse.net/cgi-bin/chadmin/viewcat/
    Health___Medicine?kywd++
http://h-devil-www.mc.duke.edu/h-devil
http://www.fitlife.com/
http://galaxy.einet.net/galaxy/Community/Health.html
http://www.cc.columbia.edu:80/cu/healthwise/
http://www.arcade.uiowa.edu/hardin-www/md.html
http://www.healthtouch.com/
http://www.healthy.net/
http://www.kidshealth.org/index2.html
http://www.northwesternmutual.com/games/longevity/
http://www.mediconsult.com/

```
http://www.ncahf.org/
http://www.aetnaushc.com/topics/index.html
http://www.stayhealthy.com/
http://www.yahoo.com/Health
http://www.youfirst.com/
```

Health and Disease Care

```
http://www.amso.com
http://www.centerwatch.com/
http://www.convergentmedical.com/
http://www.globalmedic.com/
http://www.wp.com/HCLA/
http://epn.org/idea/health.html
http://www.life-line.org/index2.html
http://www.yahoo.com/Health/Health_Care/
```

appendix

School Health Education

```
http://www.cancer.org/cshe/cshe.html
http://www.ericsp.org/
http://www.ericsp.org/hprdtoc.html
http://www.ex.ac.uk/~dregis/healthy.html
http://www.nyu.edu/education/hepr/
```

Health Promotion

```
http://www.awhp.com/
http://www.ihpr.ubc.ca/
http://www.monash.edu.au/health/
http://www.siu.edu/~crhssd/rhres.htm
http://www.welltech.com/
```

Health Psychology

```
http://www.recovery.org/aa/
http://www.apa.org/
http://www.concentric.net/~conure/allen.html
```

```
http://www.astromind.is/index.html
http://www.athealth.com/
http://www.shef.ac.uk/~psysc/psychotherapy/index.html
http://www.uwsp.edu/acad/psych/dk/danielpg.htm
http://www.coil.com/~grohol/
http://www.infinityinst.com/
http://fly.hiwaay.net/~garson/
http://www.gen.emory.edu/MEDWEB/keyword/
    mental_health~psychiatry~psychology.html
http://www.cmhc.com/
http://pie.org/E18634T3783
http://www.psyunix.iupui.edu/psych_dir.html
http://www.psych-web.com/
http://www.cloud9.net/~thorpy/
http://www.nerdworld.com/users/dstein/nw142.html
http://www.clas.ufl.edu/users/gthursby/taoism/
http://www1.rider.edu/~suler/zenstory/zenstory.html
```

Heart Health

```
http://www.americanheart.org/
http://www.cardio.com/articles/preventn.htm
http://www.cardio.com/
http://www.fi.edu/biosci/heart.html
http://sln.fi.edu/biosci/healthy/healthy.html
http://www.mindspring.com/~mtm/news.html
http://www.internetwks.com/pauling/
http://www.hsforum.com/HeartSurgery/LearningCtrHSF.html
http://www.fatfree.com/FAQ/ada-paper
```

Food and Nutrition

```
http://www.eatright.org/
http://www.amhrt.org/catalog/Health_catpage4.html
http://arborcom.com/
http://www.medlib.arizona.edu/educ/nutrition.html
http://www.dietitian.com/
http://www.holisticmed.com/aspartame/
http://www1.mhv.net/~donn/diet.html
http://www.foodwine.com/
http://www.olen.com/food/
http://www.nalusda.gov/fnic/
http://www.ganesa.com/food/index.html
http://dinnercoop.cs.cmu.edu/dinnercoop/special/health.html
```

```
http://www.envirolink.org/arrs/health_wrap.html
http://ificinfo.health.org/
http://www.mothernature.com/
http://www.mymenus.com/
http://www.nutribase.com/
http://www.vegweb.com/
```

Public Health

```
http://www.apha.org/
http://www.sph.emory.edu/studentservice/Career.html
http://www.cdc.gov/
http://www-sci.lib.uci.edu/~martindale/PHealth.html
```

Safety and Injury Prevention

appendix

```
http://www.bhsi.org/index.htm
http://www.mrg.ab.ca/christie/safelist.htm
gopher://cpsc.gov/
http://www.nsc.org/
http://www.safetylink.com/
http://vhp.nus.sg/PID/
http://www.yahoo.com/Health/Public_Health_And_Safety/
http://www.epa.gov/
```

Self-Help and Self-Care

```
http://www.enews.com/magazines/ucbwl/
http://www.healthfinder.org/default.htm
http://www.lef.org/
http://lifematters.com/index.html
http://www.hotwired.com/wired/2.01/features/healthcare.html
http://www.ns.net/~sjmoore/psites.html
http://www.gasou.edu/psychweb/resource/selfhelp.htm
http://www.lib.ox.ac.uk/internet/news/faq/archive/
    self-impr-faq.part1.html
http://www.lib.ox.ac.uk/internet/news/faq/archive/
    self-impr-faq.part2.html
http://cybertowers.com/cgibin/add_a_link.cgi?all_links=go
http://www.realtime.net/~mmjw/
```

Stress Management

```
http://www.stress.org/index.htm
http://www.algy.com/anxiety/anxiety.html
http://www.coolware.com/health/joel/stress.html
http://www.bogo.co.uk/andys/index.html
http://www.concord.wvnet.edu/~olpin/relax.html
http://www.stressfree.com/
http://imt.net/~randolfi/StressPage.html
```

Tobacco, Alcohol, and Drug Use

```
http://www.seercom.com/airspace/
http://www.Al-Anon-Alateen.org/
http://center.butler.brown.edu/
http://hyperreal.com/drugs/faqs/resources.html
http://www.jointogether.org/jto/
http://www.health.org/aboutn.htm
http://www.nida.nih.gov/
http://www.inhalants.com/
http://www.nwre.org/
http://tobacco.arizona.edu/
http://www.health.org/
http://www.cs.brown.edu/people/lsh/smoking.html
http://www.tobacco.org/
```

appendix

Violence Resources and Information

```
http://www.igc.apc.org/fund/workplace/
http://www.igc.apc.org/fund/the_facts/
http://www.execpc.com/~cpi/
http://www.cdc.gov/niosh/homepage.html
http://www.osha-slc.gov/OshDoc/Additional.html
http://venable.com/wlu/rockem.htm
```

Weight Control

http://www.dietitian.com/overweig.html
http://www.cyberdiet.com/
http://www1.mhv.net/~donn/diet.html
http://healthyweight.com/
http://www2.shapeup.org/sua/index.html
http://www.weight.com/comprehensive.html

Wellness and Optimum Health

http://www.columbia.edu/cu/healthwise/
http://www.tiac.net/users/mgold/health.html
http://www.med.harvard.edu/programs/mindbody/
http://www.wellnessnwi.org/
http://www.aboutliving.com/htmlal/index.html
http://hyperlink.com/balance

appendix

Women's Health

http://www.ivf.com/
http://www.parentsplace.com/readroom/bf.html
http://www.gen.emory.edu/medweb/medweb.gynecology.html
http://www.melpomene.org/
http://www.health-science.com/health.htm
http://www.cs.utk.edu/~bartley/saInfoPage.html
http://www1.fourlakes.net/~wha/
http://www.yahoo.com/Health/Women_s_Health/

Glossary

Your Own Private Glossary

The Glossary in this book contains reference terms you'll find useful as you get started on the Internet. After a while, however, you'll find yourself running across abbreviations, acronyms, and buzzwords whose definitions will make more sense to you once you're no longer a novice (or "newbie"). That's the time to build a glossary of your own. For now, the 2DNet Webopædia gives you a place to start.

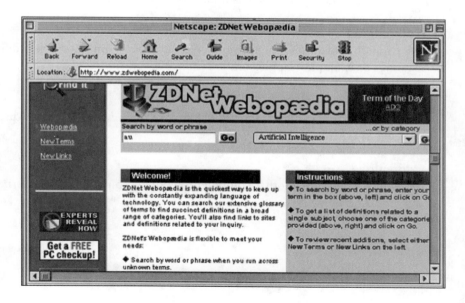

alias
A simple email address that can be used in place of a more complex one.

bandwidth
Internet parlance for capacity to carry or transfer information such as email and Web pages.

browser
The computer program that lets you view the contents of Web sites.

client
A program that runs on your personal computer and supplies you with Internet services, such as getting your mail.

DNS
See **domain name server.**

domain
A group of computers administered as a single unit, typically belonging to a single organization such as a university or corporation.

domain name
A name that identifies one or more computers belonging to a single domain. For example, "apple.com".

domain name server
A computer that converts domain names into the numeric addresses used on the Internet.

download
Copying a file from another computer to your computer over the Internet.

email
Electronic mail.

emoticon
A guide to the writer's feelings, represented by typed characters, such as the Smiley :-). Helps readers understand the emotions underlying a written message.

FAQ
Frequently Asked Questions

flame
A rude or derogatory message directed as a personal attack against an individual or group.

flame war
An exchange of flames (see above).

FTP
File Transfer Protocol, a method of moving files from one computer to another over the Internet.

home page
A page on the World Wide Web that acts as a starting point for information about a person or organization.

hypertext
Text that contains embedded *links* to other pages of text. Hypertext enables the reader to navigate between pages of related information by following links in the text.

link

A reference to a location on the Web that is embedded in the text of the Web page. Links are usually highlighted with a different color or underline to make them easily visible.

list server

Strictly speaking, a computer program that administers electronic mailing lists, but also used to denote such lists or discussion groups, as in "the writer's list server."

lurker

A passive reader of an Internet *newsgroup*. A lurker reads messages, but does not participate in the discussion by posting or responding to messages.

modem

A device for connecting two computers over a telephone line.

newbie

A new user of the Internet.

newsgroup

A discussion forum in which all participants can read all messages and public replies between the participants.

pages

All the text, graphics, pictures, and so forth, denoted by a single URL beginning with the identifier "http://".

quoted

Text in an email message or newsgroup posting that has been set off by the use of vertical bars or > characters in the left-hand margin.

search engine
A computer program that will locate Web sites or files based on specified criteria.

secure
A Web page whose contents are encrypted when sending or receiving information.

server
A computer program that moves information on request, such as a Web server that sends pages to your browser.

Smiley
See **emoticon.**

snail mail
Mail sent the old fashioned way: Write a letter, put it in an envelope, stick on a stamp, and drop it in the mailbox.

spam
Spam is to the Internet as unsolicited junk mail is to the postal system.

URL
Uniform Resource Locator: The notation for specifying addresses on the World Wide Web (e.g. http://www.abacon.com or ftp://ftp.abacon.com).

Usenet
The section of the Internet devoted to *newsgroups.*

Web site
A collection of pages administered by a single organization or individual.